HEALTH POWER

Healthy by Choice, Not by Chance!

Hans Diehl, DrHSc, MPH, FACN
Aileen Ludington, MD

Loma Linda, CA 92354

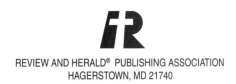

REVIEW AND HERALD® PUBLISHING ASSOCIATION
HAGERSTOWN, MD 21740

This book was
    Edited by Hans Diehl
    Cover design by Ron J. Pride
    Typeset: 11/14 Helvetica

R&H Cataloging Service

Diehl, Hans, and Aileen Ludington

    p. cm. Health Power: Healthy by Choice, Not by Chance / Hans Diehl, Aileen Ludington.
    Includes index.

    1. Health. 2. Popular Medicine. 3. Lifestyle Medicine. 4. Clinical Nutrition.   I. Diehl, Hans, 1946.
    II. Ludington, Aileen, 1926.

978-0-8280-2594-2

What Others Have Said

Clarity, Charm, and Thoroughness

"The greatest challenge of Western medicine is to educate and motivate patients to adopt a healthier lifestyle. This book is doing exactly that with clarity, charm, and thoroughness."

—William Castelli, M.D.
Former Director, Framingham Heart Study

A Solid Book

"A solid book, clearly written, providing a sensible introduction to the basis of natural health management."

—John Robbins
Author, Diet for a New America

Extend Your Life

"These are important concepts that, when internalized, will do more to improve your health and wwwextend your life than all the technological wonders of modern medicine."

—Caldwell Esselstyn, Jr., M.D.
Cleveland Clinic

No One Can Read and Remain the Same

"The authors have been in the forefront of preventive medicine since long before it was fashionable. They confront health questions and anxieties with compelling evidence and grace. No one can read even a few of these chapters and remain the same."

—Herbert E. Douglass, Th.D., former president
Weimar Institute

Most Practical Key

"This may be the most practical key to a better lifestyle that many of us have ever found."

—Dan Matthews, executive producer/host
Christian Lifestyle Magazine

Habits Count

"[Most people] suffer because of their own wrong course of action. They disregard the principles of health by their habits of eating, drinking, dressing, and working."

—E. G. White
Pioneer health reformer/educator

The Blame Game

"God is not responsible for the suffering that follows disregard of natural law."

—E. G. White
Pioneer health reformer/educator

Nature's Way

"In nature there are neither rewards nor punishments; there are only consequences."

—Robert B. Ingersoll

Can't Buy Them

"There are four things in life which money cannot buy: friends, time, peace of mind, and good health."

—William F. Kenney

Contents

Acknowledgments

CAUTION:
The information in this book is not intended to replace medical advice or treatment. Questions about symptoms and medications, general or specific, should be addressed to your physician.

We are indebted to the wholistic vision of health of the Lifestyle Medicine Institute, for believing in this project enough to extend considerable financial support and resources to see it through to completion.

In addition, we wish to give special recognition to Lawson Dumbeck, author of the *Dynamic Living Workbook*, from which the Application pages of this book are abstracted. Mr. Dumbeck is an educator and freelance writer based in Olympia, Washington. He holds graduate degrees in adult education and law.

And last, we feel greatly indebted to some 50,000 faithful graduates of our CHIP health outreach programs who continue to validate in their daily lives the principles presented in this book.

—Drs. Hans Diehl and Aileen Ludington

Preface

Consciously or unconsciously, most people make sacrifices of some sort. Unfortunately, they often sacrifice health, family, religion, or other priceless possessions in order to gain the transitory pleasures of wealth, power, status, or fame.

Imagine life as a game in which you are juggling five balls—work, family, health, friends, and religion—in the air, and you are trying to keep all of them off the ground. You will soon realize that work is a rubber ball. If you drop it, it will bounce back. But the other four balls—your family, health, friends, and spiritual life—are much more fragile. If you drop one of these, it will be scuffed, marked, nicked, damaged, or even shattered. It will never be the same again. You must understand that, and strive to balance all parts of your life.

This book will help you realize that all these aspects are largely under your control.

- Learn how you can prevent and even reverse many of today's major killer diseases.

- Learn how to make sense out of confusing and often contradictory health information, and to understand why today's breakthroughs often become tomorrow's embarrassments.

- Learn how to strengthen your social and family relationships, and cultivate a more meaningful spiritual life.

This book will help you discover—day by day and step by step—not a better life, but the best life!

Are we special?

"Sons are a heritage from the Lord, children a reward from him." —*Psalm 127:3*

Health Perspectives

Myths and Miracles

The achievements of science, medicine, and public health have been enormous. America is now an undisputed leader of quality medical care. There is much to be proud of, and more to come.

That's especially incredible considering that germs were discovered only some 150 years ago.

It has been a big jump from Louis Pasteur's discovery of the germ theory to the place we are now. His findings opened the door to antiseptic surgery, improved sanitation, cleaner water, safer food, and vaccines. All of these impacted infectious diseases, such as typhoid, cholera, poliomyelitis, and smallpox. Once a leading cause of death in developed countries, infectious diseases have now been upstaged by the noninfectious degenerative-type diseases, increasingly referred to as Western or lifestyle diseases.

What do you consider the medical landmarks of the twentieth century?

There are many. Improved surgical techniques, better anesthesia, and safer blood transfusions, for starters. Antibiotics have saved millions of lives, although their overuse is producing a frightening backlash—resistant strains of bacteria that are often unaffected by present treatments.

Advances in diagnostic technology are prodigious. The inside workings of various bodily organs can now be visualized, measured, and studied, and even thought patterns and emotions can be traced as they travel in the brain.

Molecular biology and genetics are opening doors to more new worlds.

Many birth defects can now be detected in advance, and some can be corrected in the uterus, before birth. Geneticists are learning to pinpoint predispositions to certain diseases in the DNA, and

> "Dear friend, I pray that you may enjoy good health and that all may go well with you, even as your soul is getting along well."
> —3 John 2

are looking for ways to affect the outcome.

For medical technology in the years ahead, there is no end in sight. As scientists seek to clone spare body parts from people's own cells, the limiting factors may well be cost and affordability.

No wonder people live so much longer today!

Actually that belief is largely a myth. For years people believed that the miracles of modern medicine were mainly responsible for extending our current life span by some 27 years, when compared to those who were born 100 years ago.

The fact is that around 1900 every sixth baby died before reaching the first year of life, mainly because of infectious diseases. This, then, greatly shortened the average life span of their society.

Today, however, a person age 65 has very nearly the same life expectancy as a person back then who survived that critical first year of life, with perhaps an average gain of around six or seven years at most (see graph).

Then why do we see so much more "degenerative disease"? Isn't it because most of our ancestors died while they were still too young to experience the diseases of "old age"?

The term "degenerative disease" is really a misnomer. For years people fatalistically accepted the idea that atherosclerosis-related diseases (such as coronary heart diseases and stroke), cancer, diabetes, diverticulosis, arthritis, and other ailments were diseases of old age and therefore to be expected.

Nothing could be further from the truth, because in Western society 100 years ago:

- Atherosclerosis-related diseases were virtually unknown. The first description of coronary artery disease and "heart attacks" appeared in the medical literature in 1910. Today these diseases are responsible for every third death.
- Cancers of the breast, colon, prostate, and lungs were virtually unknown. These cancers, however, are now claiming one out of every four American lives.
- Similarly, very few diabetics were known then. Yet today diabetes rates are increasing with frightening speed. (See chart on page 54.) Diabetes and its complications now represent one of the most frequent causes of death.

In light of the advances in medical science, that is truly amazing. Shouldn't these diseases be decreasing?

It's important to understand that these diseases are actually not "degenerative"—they are not necessarily the result of growing older. The fact that an increasing number of younger people are suffering from them refutes this, as does their increase to near epidemic proportions despite everything medical science can do.

Modern epidemiology (the study of disease differences in world populations) is unraveling the mystery—that most of these modern killer diseases are lifestyle-related. They are basically diseases of affluence—too much eating and drinking, too much smoking, and too little exercise.

U.S. LIFE SPAN TRENDS

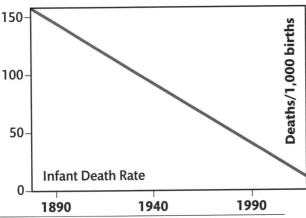

Life expectancy at birth is increasing. Life expectancy for 65-year-olds, however, has only marginally increased during the past 100 years.

Dropping the Ball

THE GOVERNMENT
What They're Doing:

The federal government shells out a mere $2 million on health and on fitness-related initiatives—some policy recommendations here, a public service campaign there.

THE MEDICAL PROFESSION
What They're Doing:

Precious little. Nearly half the people surveyed in a Gallup poll said they'd never heard a word about fitness or wellness from their doctors.

THE FITNESS INDUSTRY
What They're Doing:

Marketing the quick hit ("Thinner Thighs in 30 Days"), exercise that's painful rather than fun ("Go for the Burn"), and sexiness over health.

The Stereotypical Businessman—

overweight, exhausted, living on cigarettes and three-martini lunches—is out of date. In today's business world, sweat is status, and trimness is success. More and more modern executives are apt to be in prime condition; neither they nor their companies can afford otherwise.

Medical science is treating the symptoms, but it's time to attack the causes.

You mean people create their own diseases? You can't be serious!

Yes, I am serious. The solution to most of our health problems today does not depend on physicians, technological advances, or on the quality of our hospitals. Our health today is determined largely by our lifestyle choices, our physiological inheritance, and our physical environment. Good health in today's world mainly depends on what we're willing to do for ourselves—how we choose to live, especially how we eat, drink, exercise, and whether or not we smoke.

That's pretty scary. Yet it's good to know there are things I can do to improve my own health.

That's the bottom line. People are increasingly waking up to the fact that they must take charge of—take responsibility for—their own health. That's what this book is about. How to do it. How to live a quality life, and how to avoid the most common causes of premature disease, disability, suffering, and death. If we take advantage of the knowledge we have right now, most of us could live to be 100 in good health.

Advances in high-tech medicine have not altered the advances of the killer diseases

NOTES:

"The concept that Western diseases are lifestyle-related and therefore potentially preventable and reversible is the most important medical discovery of the twentieth century."
—Denis Burkitt, M.D., England, Discoverer of *Burkitt's Lymphoma*

The Future Shape of Healthy Living

How about you? What are some health habits you would like to work on?
Write them down in this space:

1. _____

2. _____

3. _____

4. _____

5. _____

6. _____

"Our nation's leading killer diseases are largely lifestyle related and can therefore be prevented or delayed. They are not prevented by vaccines, or cured by pills and procedures. They are largely an extension of our health damaging behaviors - our use of tobacco, lack of exercise and our rich diet."
—US Dept. Health & Human Services

From Kernel to Colonel

Americans are spending 40 percent of their food dollars eating out. Our food is processed, refined, concentrated, sugared, salted, and chemically engineered to produce taste sensations high in calories and low in nutrients. Our cattle are fattened in feedlots without exercise and with antibiotics and growth enhancers. The result: bigger cattle producing juicier steaks containing nearly twice the fat as range-fed cattle. And we are paying dearly for these advancements. While we eat to live, what we eat is killing us.

Are you saying that food can cause disease?

The statistics are pretty convincing. In 1900 fewer than 10 percent of deaths in the United States were attributed to artery disease. Today it's close to 33 percent. Back then, less than 6 percent died of cancer, while today the figure is exceeding 25 percent.

This isn't nature's way. We weren't meant to die in such numbers from heart attacks, strokes, diabetes, and from cancer of the lungs, breast, prostate, and colon. Significant cardiovascular disease (heart disease and strokes) began to emerge in America after World War I. It became rampant only after World War II, when people could afford diets rich in animal products and when the food industry began producing highly processed foods crammed with calories and emptied of nutrition. (See graph on next page)

> "This is what the kingdom of God is like. A man scatters seed on the ground. Night and day, whether he sleeps or gets up, the seed sprouts and grows, though he does not know how. All by itself the soil produces grain—first the stalk, then the head, then the full kernel in the head. As soon as the grain is ripe, he puts the sickle to it, because the harvest has come." —Mark 4:26-29

MORTALITY TRENDS FOR CVD AND CANCER (U.S. 1900-2000)

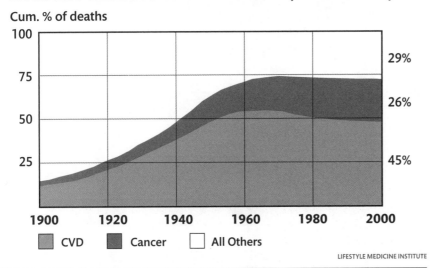

Cum. % of deaths

- CVD
- Cancer
- All Others

29%
26%
45%

LIFESTYLE MEDICINE INSTITUTE

Cardiovascular disease (CVD) and cancer (as a percentage of all causes of death) have increased over the years. While CVD at the turn of the century accounted for 10 to 15 percent of deaths, it now accounts for almost every second death. Similar increases are shown for cancer, which is continuing to rise despite heroic after-the-fact medical interventions. (U.S. 1900-2000)

Could this be coincidental?

Hardly. This problem is unique to Westernized people. Rural populations in China and Southeast Asia with little access to rich foods experience few heart attacks. Similarly, most people in rural Africa and South and Central America have little fear of diabetes and cardiovascular disease. Yet in North America, Australia, New Zealand, the increasingly affluent countries in Europe and Asia, and among the affluent in Africa, where diets are rich in fat and cholesterol, heart disease and diabetes are epidemic.

The villains—low fiber, high fat, and cholesterol—take their toll by damaging the body's vital oxygen-carrying arteries and by upsetting important metabolic functions. Because of thickened, narrowed arteries, 4,000 Americans have heart attacks every day, every third adult has high blood pressure, and thousands are crippled from strokes.

Because of disordered metabolisms from unbalanced lifestyles, obesity is epidemic, and three out of ten babies born today will develop diabetes in their lifetime.

How did these dietary changes come about?

Before 1900 the North American diet consisted mostly of foods grown in local gardens and nearby farms, supplemented with a few staples from the general store. Their meat came from barnyard animals and range-fed cattle. People then didn't have thousands of beautifully packaged and highly promoted food products waiting at the supermarket. Fast-food restaurants didn't beckon from nearly every street corner.

The backbone of their diet was kernels—kernels of wheat and other grains growing in reassuring profusion. Families ate freshly cooked food and thick slices of home-baked bread around their own tables. They enjoyed hot cereals, cornbread, and biscuits. They ate rice, pasta, and corn, along with beans, potatoes, vegetables, and fruit. These nutri-

Fruits, Vegetables, Grains, Legumes

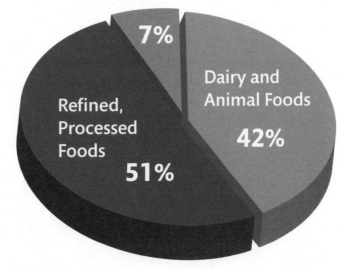

7%

Dairy and Animal Foods 42%

Refined, Processed Foods 51%

USDA Agriculture Fact Book, 2010

Calories consumed from different foods by source.

Refined Foods

Food "as grown" is nutritionally balanced. Refinement, however, strips food of most of its fiber and nutrients. Processing adds calories, subtracts nutrition, and contributes myriads of chemical additives.

Protein Changes

In 1900, Americans got 70% of their protein from plant foods. Today, they get 70% of their protein from animal product—high in fat and cholesterol and devoid of fiber.

DIETARY TRENDS *(in % of total calories)*

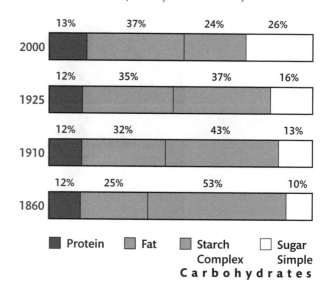

| Protein | Fat | Starch Complex | Sugar Simple |
| | | Complex | Simple |

Carbohydrates

The standard American diet (SAD) has been shifting, resulting in a dramatic change in its composition. Today more calories come from sugar (simple carbohydrates) than from starch (complex carbohydrates) and more than one third of the calories come from fat. (U.S. 1860-2000)

That's frightening! What can be done?

Education is the key. As people learn that refinement robs food of most of its fiber and nutrients, and processing adds calories, subtracts nutrition, and contributes scores of chemical additives, many are willing to make changes.

People are also realizing that meat and dairy products should be used sparingly. While they carry nutrients, most of them are too high in fat, cholesterol, animal protein, and calories. And often they are loaded with hormones and pesticides, and they contain virtually no fiber.

Intelligent people are increasingly giving up their preoccupation with rich animal products and processed foods. Instead, they are eating more unrefined complex carbohydrates—whole plant foods, usually rich in fiber.

Many people know it, and science confirms it. The road to better health and longer life detours around fast-food outlets, feedlot animals, and shops full of contrived and depleted foods. Instead, the road to better health leads back to the gardens and farmlands—to the fresh fruits and crisp vegetables, and to the kernels of golden grain.

tious high-fiber foods then made up 53 percent of their daily calorie intake. (See graph)

Last year Americans grew almost 10 billion bushels of corn—but less than 1 percent of this crop was sweet corn, the kind we eat as a vegetable. The rest was used for animal feed, soft drinks (high fructose corn syrup, corn chips, gasoline additives, and paper.) But times and tastes have changed dramatically. Cereals like oatmeal have been replaced by cold, presweetened flakes. Lunch typically consists of a salad soaked in oily dressing, a hamburger, and a soda. And dinner often comes frozen in a cardboard box or from the colonel. Between meals there are sodas, chips, Ding Dongs, and doughnuts. Nutritious, unrefined high fiber foods, such as fruits, vegetables, grains and legumes, now represent only 7 percent of our daily calories. The clear majority of calories today comes from refined, processed foods (51%) and dairy and animal foods (42%). (See graph on previous page.)

Some 100 years ago very few Americans suffered from coronary heart disease, stroke, and cancer. Today these lifestyle-related diseases account for the majority of deaths in North America. The good news is that you don't have to become a statistic. By adopting a simpler diet and wiser lifestyle habits, you can live longer and enjoy a healthier, more productive life.

The Choice Is Yours

You Can Do It

Simply eating a simple, more traditional diet of foods as grown and walking at least 10,000 steps a day offer you the same freedom from coronary heart disease, stroke, diabetes, and cancer that your ancestors enjoyed. It's possible. You need three essentials.

The Three Essentials

Desire: To modify a habit, you must want to change. Established patterns are comfortable. To break their grip, you need a strong desire to energize yourself.

Knowledge: Desire alone can't change entrenched lifestyle patterns. You must also know what to change and understand why you should change it.

For instance, although most people want to avoid clogged arteries, achieving this is impossible without a knowledge of the harmful effects of excess cholesterol and fat in the diet.

Skill: Just knowing what to do isn't enough. You need to know how to do it. And then you need to practice it until the new behavior becomes automatic.

Skills that promote health include learning how to cook cholesterol-free, low-fat meals, developing a program of regular exercise, reading food labels to avoid highly salted products, and becoming skilled at choosing more natural, traditional food at food outlets.

Try this simple experiment. Eat one or two servings of fresh fruit every morning for the next three weeks. Eat as many different kinds as you can find.

Your Fresh Fruit List:

Write them down in this space

1. _____
   _____
2. _____
   _____
3. _____
   _____
4. _____
   _____
5. _____
   _____

Seven Wrong Roads

As Americans, we pride ourselves on being the best-fed nation on earth. But we are paying a high price for the privilege—in needless disease, disability, and premature death.

What are we doing wrong?

Americans are eating too much of nearly everything—too much sugar, too much fat, too much cholesterol, and too much salt. We eat too many calories. And we eat too often.

Such abundance has helped lay the foundation for coronary artery disease, stroke, high blood pressure, arthritis, adult-onset diabetes, obesity, and several kinds of cancer. These diseases are responsible for three out of four deaths. They are related to our lifestyle, especially to how we eat.

Disease from food? You must mean pesticides and preservatives!

Surprisingly, pesticides and preservatives aren't the worst offenders. Here are some of the more serious culprits:

1. **Sugar**
   The National Research Council reports that refined sugars and sweeteners account for up to 20 percent of many people's daily calories. Devoid of fiber and nutrients, refined sugars are empty, or naked, calories. But because of their caloric density, they are well suited to promote obesity.

2. **Refined Foods**
   People used to think refinement was good because it got rid of useless roughage. Now we're learning how necessary fiber is in protecting us from certain cancers, stabilizing blood sugar, controlling weight, and preventing gastrointestinal problems, such as gallstones, hemorrhoids, diverticulitis, and constipation.

Many of us are digging our own graves with fork and knife.

"He who guards his mouth and his tongue keeps himself from calamity." —Proverbs 21:23

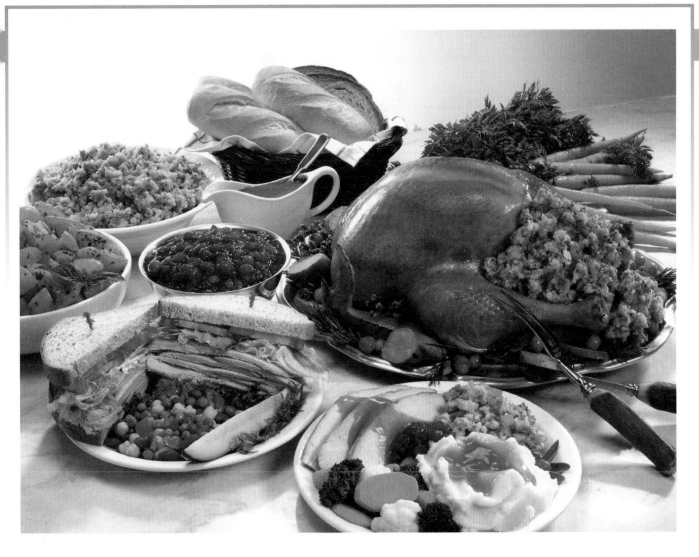

3. **Salt**

Most Westerners consume in excess of 10 grams (two teaspoons) of salt a day. This is 10 times more than is actually needed and contributes prominently to high blood pressure, heart failure, and kidney disease.

4. **Fat**

Most people don't realize that they are consuming two to three times more fat, oil, and grease than is optimal for good health. As a result, blood vessels plug up, impotence sets in, and hearts and brains suffer. A high-fat diet also contributes to overweight, adult diabetes, and certain cancers.

5. **Protein**

A diet heavy in meat and animal products provides more protein, fat, and cholesterol than the body can use. Westerners eat twice

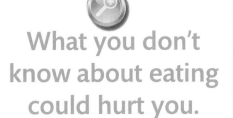

What you don't know about eating could hurt you.

as much protein than is recommended. Scientists now recognize that a more natural, traditional diet containing less animal protein and much less fat and

cholesterol is essential for improved health and longevity. (See graph next page.)

6. **Beverages**

North Americans don't drink enough water. Instead, they average several servings of soda pop, beer, coffee, tea, and sweet drinks every day. Because most of these drinks are loaded with calories from sugar and alcohol, they can play havoc with blood sugar levels and sabotage weight-control efforts. Caffeine, phosphates, and other chemicals found in beverages pose additional health risks.

7. **Snacks**

Engineered taste sensations are

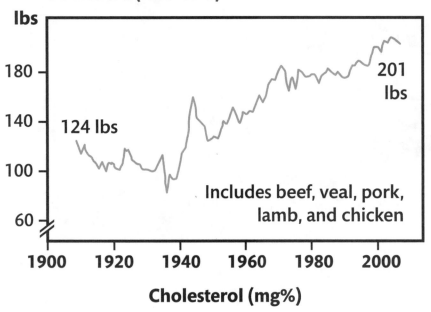

MEAT CONSUMPTION (lbs/capita)
US TRENDS (1909-2009)

124 lbs

201 lbs

Includes beef, veal, pork, lamb, and chicken

Cholesterol (mg%)

N Barnard, 2010 USDA, Econ. Res. Service

good diet and a gold mine of delectable and healthful foods. And add a few nuts every day.

Eating a variety of whole plant foods will furnish all the fat, protein, fiber, and nutrients the body needs. It's also ecologically sensitive and will cut your food budget in half.

The best news is that this kind of dietary lifestyle helps delay, arrest, and reverse and often prevents the onset of most Western killer diseases. Eating full-fiber plant foods not only allows people to eat larger quantities of food without having to worry about weight gain, but also can promote optimum health and energy for a lifetime.

taking the place of real food. It has become fashionable for schools, day-care centers—even hospitals—to make snacks available. The coffee break has become the standard at work, and snacks reign supreme after school and at home. Well-planned family meals are now the exception. Snack attacks disrupt digestion, overburden the stomach, and are a frequent cause of bloating and indigestion.

Is there anything *safe* to eat?

Think fruit—almost endless varieties, spectacular colors, and every imaginable texture and flavor. Go for vegetables, potatoes, and yams. Include legumes—all kinds of beans, lentils, chickpeas—in scores of shapes, colors, and flavors. And don't forget the grains, such as whole wheat, brown rice, and oats, which are the mainstay of a

Master Healer

But the Master Healer never passed by a human being as worthless, and we can't either. With a restored sense of self-worth, we become willing to take risks. And taking risks in loving others is what life is all about.

NOTES:

Too much! Too much sugar! Too many refined foods! Too much salt, fat, protein, beverages, and snacks in our diet. It's a deadly mix. Only by eating less of these substances and eating more whole plant foods can we enjoy optimum health and energy.

Is There Too Much on Our Plate?

A "Fat Tooth"?

Americans eat too much fat, oil, and grease, and they pay for it with heart attacks, strokes, obesity, and other diseases.

Slim Your Salad Down

Four tablespoons of regular blue cheese or ranch dressing adds more than 500 calories to a salad.

That is 500 calories you don't need. This week, try your salads with lemon, or mix up some super salad dressing using this recipe:

Super Salad Dressing

1/4 c water
1/4 tsp Italian seasoning
1/4 tsp garlic powder
1/4 c lemon juice
1/4 tsp onion powder
1/4 tsp salt (optional)

Combine all ingredients and shake well. Let it sit; it'll get even better with age.

Write the letter of the correct description in each blank.

____ Sugar   ____ Snacks   ____ Fat

____ Salt   ____ Protein   ____ Beverages   ____ Refined Foods

A. Americans consume these instead of water. Most are loaded with calories and chemicals.

B. Fiber protects us from certain cancers, stabilizes blood sugar, and helps control our weight. It is difficult to find in these foods.

C. North Americans eat up to 10 times more than they really need. It contributes to high blood pressure, heart failure, and kidney disease.

D. Many people get close to 40 percent of their daily calories from this. It plugs up arteries and contributes to overweight and Type II diabetes.

E. It makes up more than 20 percent of America's daily calories, yet provides no fiber or nutrients.

F. Americans eat twice as much of this than is recommended. Scientists now recognize that too much can be harmful.

G. These often take the place of real food. They are low in nutrition, high in price, and can disrupt digestion.

Growing Healthy Kids

Remember the simple pleasures of just being a kid?

The news is not good. "Heart disease begins in childhood," reports the National Institutes of Health. A recent examination of 360 randomly selected youngsters ages 7 to 12 revealed that 98 percent of the children already had three or more risk factors for heart disease.

But we keep hearing that people are getting healthier!

It's mainly the grown-ups who are exercising, losing weight, quitting tobacco, and becoming more health-conscious.

But it's a different story for kids. "Since the early 1960s the general health of adolescents has declined," says the American Academy of Pediatrics. "And it has been escalating over the last 25 years. Today's kids are flabby. They don't have the proper cardiovascular tone. They are not physically fit."

Too much television?

Television certainly has had an impact. Time spent in front of the TV set is time taken away from body building, calorie-burning physical activities such as running, bicycling, skating, basketball, or climbing trees. That sets the stage for excessive weight gain, which in itself is a risk factor for high blood cholesterol and heart disease.

Exercise physiologist Kate O'Shea warns that "the junior couch potato of today is the fat farm candidate of tomorrow."

Don't school physical education programs help?

Only a few schools require students to take physical education in all grades. In an era of tight budgets and teacher shortages, health and physical education programs are often among the first to go.

What about children's eating habits?

With nine out of 10 Saturday-morning food advertisements on

"Train a child in the way he should go, and when he is old he will not turn from it." —Proverbs 22:6

the networks hawking processed foods, high in sugar, fat, and salt, television significantly influences the food preferences of children from their earliest years.

Home-cooked, sitting-down-around-the-table meals are now the exception in most American homes, being largely replaced by fast foods and engineered foods. More than half of today's high school kids head off to fast-food chains and snack machines instead of school lunch rooms.

Any good news?

The good news is that children can be taught—and the younger they get started, the better.

Here are some tips for building

A body is a terrible thing to waste.

good health habits early in life:
- Daily exercise—preferably out-doors—for at least an hour.
- Three meals a day, at regular times, with lots of whole grains, legumes, fruits, and vegetables. Discourage snacks, and the child will have a better appetite for nutritious food at mealtimes. If a snack is needed, offer a piece of fresh fruit.
- Push plenty of water. Save sodas for special occasions.
- Control TV. The hours a child watches TV relate directly to weight gain and elevated blood cho-lesterol levels.
- Adequate rest. Most children are chronically tired—not surprising

How to raise GOOD kids

- Be good parents; set the example.
- Maintain consistent united discipline.
- Clearly explain boundaries and expectations.
- Teach responsibility early.
- Let children work for money.
- Have a good attitude toward your kids.
- Think positive with them.
- Teach spiritual values.
- Have fun together.
- Learn to listen—really listen.
- Give them unconditional love.

NOTES

when you remember that teenagers do best on nine hours of sleep a night, and younger ones need more. Put the kids to bed early enough so they awaken naturally in time for a healthy breakfast

- Cultivate a wide range of interests—schedule library visits, music lessons, arts and crafts, hobbies, and family outings. Children who spend time with their parents and develop deep spiritual roots experience less stress and improved mental health.
- Set a good example. The life choices you are modeling day by day are the strongest determinants of your children's future behavior.

Is it worth the effort?

"Fitness can be fun," says Arnold Schwarzenegger, who was President George H. W. Bush's spokesman for the Council on Physical Fitness and Sports. "Stay away from junk food. Get off the couch. Unplug the Nintendo. Turn off the TV. Go out and get some exercise! A body is a terrible thing to waste."

Application

Time spent with children encourages greater trust and better communication. Teaching and modeling spiritual values deepens spiritual roots. Children need these basics to cope with the stresses of growing up into balanced, mentally healthy adults.

How many things can you think of that will help relationships with the children in your life?

Write them down in this space:

1. _____

   _____

2. _____

   _____

3. _____

   _____

4. _____

   _____

5. _____

   _____

6. _____

   _____

7. _____

   _____

   _____

Older Can Be Better

Everyone hates getting old. People want to stay young or at least middle-aged. But time keeps marching. With the 65-and-older segment getting larger in North America, what are the prospects for the golden-agers in today's world?

An increasing trend is to date people by their intellectual and social capabilities rather than by chronological age. Health, rather than years, usually determines one's status. Old age sets in when disease and disability limit everyday tasks. Some people are old while still relatively young in years. These are usually people who are chronically ill, injured, or victims of a major tragedy, many of whom withdraw and give up on life. Others remain youthful, vital, interesting, and productive into advanced age.

Some people claim older is better. Can that be?

It's a matter of perspective. For physical strength, energy and fewer ailments, youth is better. But for increased confidence, better judgment and insight, less anxiety, and more freedom, older can be better. And experience helps too. Most philosophers, composers, painters, and writers, for instance, improve with time.

Don't most people over 65 suffer from chronic illnesses?

In affluent Western society, about 80 percent of the 65-and-over group have some kind of health problem, such as high blood pressure, arthritis, diabetes, depression, or heart disease. But most of these illnesses are not incapacitating. About 95 percent of older people live in their communities, and most have their own households.

Premature aging and disability are largely the result of lifestyle factors, such as smoking, excessive alcohol and caffeine consumption, and the abuse of drugs. Being overweight speeds up physical and sexual decline. A diet of rich, refined foods and lack of regular exercise can make people old before their time.

You've seen 10 presidents and a man on the moon. Now go see your grandchildren!

"Grandchildren are the crown of the elderly."
—Proverbs 17:6, Clear Word

Isn't forgetfulness a bad sign?

Forgetfulness in older people is exaggerated. Stress, anxiety, fast-moving events, memory overload, and lack of interest can cause forgetfulness at any age. Depression, which affects many older people, is often misdiagnosed as senility. Not too many actually develop genuinely senile dementias. Most people retain remarkable memory function for a long time, especially when they stay active and fit.

Don't many older people end up in nursing homes?

Actually, in North America only 2 percent of people 64 to 75 years of age live in nursing homes.

Research shows that a healthy lifestyle can hold back the aging process as much as 30 years.

Only after age 85 does the figure reach 20 percent.

Today is a good time to be alive! Productive social activities are pushing back the aging process. So are exercise, a better understanding of the role of diet, earlier attention to health problems, and advances in modern technology. People today are often staying physically and mentally fit into their 80s and 90s. Many remain sexually active as well.

There is more. Scientists are dis-

It's true—many things get better with age.

Beautiful young people are accidents of nature. Beautiful old people are works of art.

covering that an optimistic, positive attitude actually boosts the body's immune mechanism. This sophisticated defense system is proving to be one of the major keys to good health.

The Good Book said it long ago: "A merry heart does good, like medicine" (Proverbs 17:22, NKJV).

NOTES

A diet of rich, refined foods and a lack of exercise can make you old before your time. But with a healthy lifestyle, worthwhile goals, and a positive mental attitude, it is possible to enjoy life well into your golden years.

Super Seniors!

Hulda Crooks, at age 66, decided to take on a new challenge—mountain climbing. Over the next 25 years she scaled some of North America's tallest peaks, plus Mount Fuji, the tallest mountain in Japan.

Bob Andersen would drive to the mailbox rather than walk the 50 yards it took to pick up his mail. Then he settled for simpler foods and a daily exercise. And two years later, at the age of 68, he bicycled more than 2,000 miles across Canada in 60 days.

"The second childhood certainly beats the first, because there's no one around to tell you what you can't do."
—Bob Andersen

What's in Your Future?

Take a moment to imagine yourself on your 90th birthday. Are you standing atop a mountain? painting a picture? celebrating life with family and friends? Or are you ill and isolated?

A positive attitude is important for physical health and happiness. Without purpose, goals, and productive social activities, we age quickly. Do you have interests and goals that will carry you through your lifetime?

List three interests or goals you would like to pursue. Is there something you've always wanted to try? Someplace you wanted to visit? Something you hoped to contribute?

1. _____
_____

2. _____
_____

3. _____
_____

Choose one of the goals you've listed. If you were going to pursue it, what would be the first steps you would take?

1. _____
_____

2. _____
_____

3. _____
_____

Want to enjoy the "good life" with good health?

MODERN MEDICINE has made great strides. But some of the greatest strides have been found to relate back to rather simple things: what you eat, what you drink, what you think, and what you do.

Diseases of Lifestyle

- Coronary Heart Disease
- Reversing Heart Disease
- Hypertension
- Stroke
- Cancer
- Diabetes
- Osteoporosis
- Arthritis
- Obesity
- Alcohol
- Tobacco-related Diseases
- Caffeine Addiction
- Legalized Drug Abuse

"Don't you know that you yourselves are God's temple and that God's Spirit lives in you?"
—1 Corinthians 3:16

Killer for Dinner

H undreds of thousands of people die every year from heart attacks without a murmur of protest from the public, the press, or government agencies. Yet the nation's number one killer can be found right on the American dinner table!

Do you mean that what we eat causes heart attacks?

Yes, but not everything. The main culprits are excessive amounts of fat and cholesterol. The underlying problem is narrowing, hardening, and, eventually, plugging up of vital arteries that supply the heart with oxygen. The process is known as atherosclerosis.

People are born with clean, flexible arteries. They should stay that way throughout life. The arteries of many North Americans, however, are clogging up with cholesterol, fat, and calcium—a concoction that gradually hardens and eventually chokes off needed oxygen supplies.

During World War II most Europeans were forced to change their eating habits from their customary diet of meat, eggs, and dairy products to a more austere diet of potatoes, grains, beans, roots, and vegetables. The result? A dramatic decrease in atherosclerosis-related diseases, such as heart attacks, strokes, diabetes, gallstones, as well as certain cancers and arthritis. The marked drop in the rates of these diseases was felt for as long as 15 years after World War II.

Since then, massive amounts of data have accumulated from research on animals and humans around the world. The results are essentially the same: diets high in fat and cholesterol produce elevated levels of blood cholesterol and heart disease by clogging up the coronary arteries. Diets low in fat and cholesterol reduce blood cholesterol levels and heart disease by opening up the diameter of these arteries.

How can I tell if I have atherosclerosis?

There simply aren't any hints of the problem until your arteries are seriously narrowed, or they plug up with a sudden plaque breakoff.

> *"Heart disease before age 80 is our fault. It's not God's fault, or nature's will."*
> —*Paul Dudley White, M.D.*

> **"Above all else, guard your heart, for it is the wellspring of life."**
> —Proverbs 4:23

Some people begin to experience angina (heart pain) on exertion. For many people a heart attack is the first sign of trouble. About one third of heart attacks result in sudden death.

Who is at risk for a heart attack?

The famous Farmingham study has taught us that the risk factor concept is a good way to determine the likelihood of coronary heart disease:

- The most serious risk factor by far is an elevated blood cholesterol. Men, 50 years and older, with cholesterol levels over 295 mg% (or 7.6 mmol/L) are 10 times more likely to develop atherosclerosis than men the same age with levels under 200 mg% (or 5.1 mmol/L). A 20 percent decrease in blood cholesterol levels lowers the risk of a coronary by 50 percent.
- By age 60, smokers are 10 times more likely than non-smokers to die from heart disease. More than 160,000 coronary deaths a year are directly related to smoking, about 30 percent of the total.
- In North America every third adult has high blood pressure. This triples the likelihood of coronary death when compared to a person with normal blood pressure.
- Obese men are five times more likely to die of heart disease by age 60 than men of normal weight.
- Other risk factors are diabetes,

elevated triglycerides, sedentary lifestyle, stress, and possibly an elevated homocysteine blood level. Fortunately, all of these risk factors can be controlled by changes in diet and lifestyle. Heredity, age, and gender are risk factors a person cannot control, but they are usually the least important ones (*see graph*).

Four thousand times a day someone in the U.S. has a heart attack.

What about medications and surgery?

For those with dangerous cholesterol levels that do not respond adequately to diet, medications may be needed. Medications, however, are expensive. Furthermore, most have serious side effects. They require fre-

quent laboratory tests and physician checkups.

More glamorous are the surgical procedures: bypass operations, roto-rooter cleanouts, balloon stretching, and stenting. Some results have been spectacular. But as time goes on and statistics accumulate, it is becoming apparent that most of these operations do not prolong life or even necessarily improve it. Medical treatment is temporary at best. The only long-term solution is a serious lifestyle change.

So what is the best approach?

It is always better to prevent than to repair. But if heart disease has developed, as suggested by the presence of coronary risk factors and documented by diagnostic tests, it still isn't too late to make lifestyle changes. You can actually clean out your arteries, lower your risk of dying of atherosclerosis, and extend your active, productive years. You can markedly change your risk fac-

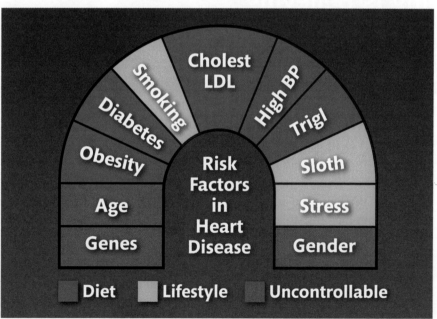

The higher on the arch, the higher the contribution of the risk factor to heart disease. Five of the eight controllable risk factors are largely under the control of diet.

CORONARY HEART DISEASE

PROGRESSION OF CORONARY ARTERY DISEASE

AGE   10   20   40   60   70

"People in Framingham with cholesterol levels below 150 mg% had no heart attacks."

—William Castelli, M.D., reporting on the famous Framingham Heart Study

tors no matter how old you are, often in just a few weeks.

Start with healthful, home-cooked meals that are very low in fat and cholesterol, yet high in unrefined complex carbohydrates and fiber. Such a diet can lower elevated cholesterol levels by 15 to 25 percent and reverse many cases of diabetes in less than four weeks (see page 52). When combined with salt restriction, this diet will also help normalize blood pressure and control obesity (see pages 40 and 64).

Begin an active daily exercise program.

If Americans would lower their cholesterol to below 180 and their blood pressures to under 125 mmHg and quit smoking, it has been estimated that 82 percent of all heart attacks before age 65 could be prevented. Simple changes in lifestyle would do more to improve the health of our nation than all the hospitals, surgeries, and drugs put together.

Seeing Is Believing . . .

This *HeartScreen* test will help you identify and understand your own risk factors, and guide you in dealing with them. It will approximate your relative risk and will help you identify areas that you may want to work on. In this test, eight risk factors are listed, and scores from 1 to 8 are assigned to each factor.

HeartScreen: Interpreting Your Score

0-6   IDEAL—Development of heart disease or stroke is extremely unlikely, especially if your cholesterol level is below 160.

7-14   ELEVATED—The development of heart disease or stroke is about one third of the U.S. average, yet three times higher than for the ideal group.

15-22   HIGH RISK—This is the average. You cannot afford to be average, because your risk is 10 times higher than the ideal group.

23-30   VERY HIGH RISK—The development of heart disease and stroke is about three times the U.S. average, or 30 times higher than the ideal group. Action is imperative! You may be able to drop four points on this test within four to eight weeks by lowering cholesterol and blood pressure through dietary change.

31-40   DANGEROUS—The likelihood of having a heart attack or stroke is about four to six times the U.S. average and about 50 times higher than the ideal group. Set goals and take action without delay!

Coronary Heart Disease—Are You at Risk?

HEARTSCREEN SELF-SCORING TEST OF HEART ATTACK AND STROKE RISK

Risk Factor	Risk Level and Score								
	0	1	2	3	4	5	6	7	8
1. Cholesterol* (mg%)**	under 160	160-179	180-199	200-219	220-239	240-259	260-279	280-299	300+
2. Blood Pressure* (mmHg)	under 110	110-119	120-129	130-139	140-149	150-159	160+		
3. Smoking (cig./day)	none	up to 5	5-9	10-19	20-29	30-39	40+		
4. Overweight† (in %)	0-4	5-9	10-14	15-19	20-29	30+			
5. Triglycerides* *** (mg%)	under 100	100-149	150-249	250-349	350+				
6. Diabetes (duration in years)	none	under 5	5-10	10+					
7. Resting Pulse (beats/min.)	under 56	56-62	63-69	70-80	80+				
8. Stress	rarely tense	tense 3x/wk	tense 2-3/day	tense and rushed	on tran-quilizers				

Risk Factor Score

1. Cholesterol ___
2. Blood Pressure ___
3. Smoking ___
4. Overweight ___
5. Triglycerides ___
6. Diabetes ___
7. Pulse ___
8. Stress ___

Total Score: ___

* To determine your cholesterol, triglycerides, and blood pressure, just see your physician. The blood test is very simple and inexpensive, and takes about five minutes. What you learn may save your life! If you take blood pressure pills, score four points regardless of your blood pressure level.

† To determine your percentage of overweight, look up your ideal weight (see p. 169), take its midpoint, and subtract it from your actual weight. Divide the difference in pounds by your ideal weight and multiply by 100.

** To convert to mmol/L divide by 39

*** To convert to mmol/L divide by 89

Eat Your Way Out

The sports world rejoiced when former Yale president Bart Giamotti became commissioner of baseball. A few months later a shocked nation wept when this respected man died suddenly at age 51, attacked by his heart.

Listed as one of the 100 most influential people in the world, Tim Russert, America's beloved and respected television journalist, appeared for 16 years as the longest-serving moderator of NBC's *Meet the Press*. In April of 2008, he performed well on his doctor's stress test. Two months later, on June 13, at the age of 58, an important irreplacable voice in American journalism had been silenced by an unexpected heart attack.

Scenarios like these are repeated thousands of times each day across North America. Heart disease now strikes a deadly blow to three out of every 10 Americans.

Is there no way out? Does it have to be like this?

Yes ... and no.

As long as Americans continue to eat their rich, fatty diet, the statistics will remain the same. We've known for years that a diet high in fat and cholesterol is the primary and essential cause of coronary heart disease. But there is a way out. We have to eat less fat, oil, and grease, and cut back on our cholesterol intake. To the extent that we commit to do this, we can help prevent and even reverse heart disease.

Despite subhuman diets and torture, survivors of the Holocaust were surprisingly free of atherosclerosis. It was the first indication— later confirmed by angiographic examinations of American POWs in Vietnam—that the process of atherosclerosis is reversible. Those held longest in captivity had the cleanest arteries.

Are you saying that heart disease may be curable?

It looks more and more that way.

The idea took on a life of its own when a young cardiologist, Dr. Dean Ornish, published a report in the *Lancet* medical journal, in 1990, that shook up the medical community. Dr. Ornish spent one year studying 48 men with advanced heart disease, many of whom were candidates for coronary bypass surgery.

He randomly assigned the men to two groups. Both groups were asked to quit smoking and to walk daily. In addition, the first group practiced stress management and followed a strict vegetarian diet with less than 10 percent of their calories coming from fat and with virtually no cholesterol.

The second group was given the standard American Heart Association's "Prudent Diet" for heart disease. This diet allowed 30 percent of calories as fat and up to 300 milligrams of cholesterol a day. At the end of the year, when the results were presented at the Scientific Session of

the American Heart Association in Washington, D.C., they became front-page news all over America.

Dr. Ornish reported that those on the very-low-fat vegetarian diet not only dropped their dangerous LDL-cholesterol levels by 37 percent, but 82 percent of their narrowed, plaque-filled arteries had actually widened, allowing more blood and oxygen to nourish the heart muscle. The heart disease had, in fact, begun to reverse itself. And the older men

with the most advanced disease actually had the best results.

The group on the so-called Prudent Diet, however, had virtually no cholesterol drop, and most of their coronary arteries showed increased narrowing— their heart disease had actually gotten worse.

You mean the American Heart Association's diet did not help at all?

Their Prudent Diet, designed for the prevention and treatment of heart disease, did not do its job. At the press conference Dr. Ornish concluded:

"The moderate diet recommendations of the American Heart Association do not go far enough to effectively influence the progression

Keys to Reversing Heart Disease

It may be the nation's leading cause of death, but it needn't be yours. And you can actually reverse it!

1. Reduce blood cholesterol to less than 160 mg% (4.1 mmol/L) with a very-low-fat, high-fiber vegetarian diet, and with cholesterol-lowering medication, if necessary.

2. Lose weight by eating more foods-as-grown and fewer refined foods and animal products.

3. Drop your high blood pressure by cutting the salt to less than five grams (or 5,000 milligrams) a day, and by getting into a daily exercise program.

4. Stop smoking and reduce alcohol intake. Alcohol is toxic to a struggling heart.

REVERSING HEART DISEASE

Patient, Heal Thyself!

Outside of on-the-job hazards, the biggest threat to the health of employees is their own lifestyle. Studies have convincingly demonstrated that a rich diet, sedentary living, drinking, and smoking largely determine the risk for developing heart disease, stroke, diabetes, cirrhosis of the liver, and cancer of the lungs, breast, colon, and prostate.

of coronary heart disease. People with clinically demonstrated disease need to go beyond the present dietary recommendation."

In another study, commenced in 1985, Caldwell Esselstyn, Jr, MD, a well-known surgeon at the famous Cleveland Clinic, took 18 patients with established, serious coronary artery disease and instructed them to follow a very strict whole foods diet very low in fats, oil and grease. Refined foods and animal products were not allowed. Within weeks, their blood cholesterol levels dropped dramatically below 160 mg% (4.1 mmol/L), where they remained over the next 20 years.

What was the clinical outcome of this strict dietary study?

1. Prior to joining the dietary experiment, these 18 coronary patients had suffered 49 cardiovascular events (such as angina and heart attacks, strokes, bypass surgeries, angioplasties) over a period of 8 years with cholesterol levels around 230 (5.9) while under excellent cardiological care at the Cleveland Clinic. In his 12-year

follow up report in the American Journal of Cardiology, Dr. Esserlstyn showed zero cardiovascular events!

2. Dr. Esselstyn was able to document angiographically that atherosclerotic plaque had consistently not only been halted and arrested but reversed. His documented 20 to 30% regression facilitated an often dramatically improved blood flow to the heart muscle which, in general, alleviated angina pain and reduced the need for angina medication. His 20 year follow-up findings have been published in his 2007 book *Prevent and Reverse Heart Disease*.

We have known for years that much of today's coronary heart disease could be prevented. But it's exciting to realize that, under the proper conditions, it is now also possible to reverse it. This revolutionary study suggests that, given the proper diet, we may be able to eat ourselves out of heart disease.

Despite subhuman diets and torture, survivors of the Holocaust were surprisingly free of atherosclerosis. It was the first indication—later confirmed by angiographic examinations of American POWs in Vietnam—that the process of atherosclerosis is reversible. Those held longest in captivity had the cleanest arteries.

NOTES

We are born with clean, flexible arteries, but excessive fat and cholesterol in the diet can clog them. Eventually this chokes off the oxygen supply to vital organs. The highly respected intervention studies by Dean Ornish, MD, and Caldwell Esselstyn MD, established the concept that plaque-filled arteries in patients who changed to a very-low-fat vegetarian diet actually began to open up. This allowed more blood and oxygen to the heart and other vital organs, and drastically reduced their angina pain.

A Killer on the Loose

Heart attacks are the leading cause of death in North America—and too much fat is the leading cause of heart attacks. This is especially true for the saturated fat (mostly coming from animal sources) and for the partially hydrogenated trans fats. Isn't it time you reduced the amount you are eating?

Getting the Fat Out

Here are four general strategies you can use to reduce the fat in your diet.

Substitute: If you use milk, then drink skim milk instead of whole milk. Or, better yet, use a non-dairy substitute. Try a bowl of chilled fruit instead of ice cream for dessert. Look for healthful substitutes for the high-fat items in your diet, such as cheeses, meats, dressings, and oils.

Reduce: Instead of ordering an eight-ounce steak, try a smaller portion with pasta or a vegetarian lasagna. Instead of a whole piece of pie, take just a sliver. Eat smaller portions of your favorite high-fat foods. This allows you to savor a few decadent bites while still cutting fat from your diet.

Eliminate: Eliminate as many temptations as possible. If you don't buy it and bring it into the house, you won't eat it.

Eliminate high-fat foods. It can work wonders. In the headline-making studies of Drs. Ornish and Esselstyn, the subjects who reversed the narrowing in their arteries were those who had reduced milk or eliminated meat and dairy products entirely.

Construct: Processed foods are stuffed with added fat. If you want to regain control over what goes into your body, cook for yourself. Get a good low-fat cookbook for educational resources and learn how to prepare delicious new dishes. It's the surest way to protect yourself from the deadly effects of too much fat.

Get Started!

List some specific ways you can apply the principles of substitution, reduction, elimination, and construction to your diet:

Substitute:

_____

_____

Reduce:

_____

_____

Eliminate:

_____

_____

Construct:

_____

The Silent Killer

Every third adult in North America has high blood pressure. These hypertensives are three times more likely to have a heart attack, five times more likely to develop heart failure, and eight times more likely to suffer a stroke than people with normal blood pressure.

How can I know if I have hypertension?

Hypertension is defined as a systolic blood pressure reading (the top number) consistently over 130, and/or a diastolic (lower number) reading of 85 or above. The optimal level is now below 120/80. Even though high blood pressure has no symptoms (that's why it's called the silent disease), it can cause progressive changes in the blood vessels until the first sign hits, usually a stroke or a heart attack.

What causes the blood pressure to go up?

Certain kinds of tumors will do it; also diseases within the kidney itself. But in 90 percent of everyday hypertension, no specific organic causes can be determined. It's for this reason that this common kind of hypertension is called *essential hypertension*.

The following factors contribute to essential hypertension:

- ***High Salt/Sodium Intake.*** Surprisingly, hypertension is uncommon in populations whose salt intake is very low. In countries with high salt intake, however (as in Japan), the disease is epidemic. Americans consume, on average, in excess of 10 grams of salt per day. That's over two teaspoonsful, or about 10 times the amount of salt that the body actually needs! And it's the

Sodium is essential for body metabolism. But too much can cause trouble. Excess sodium can stay in body tissues and hold extra water. This causes swelling, which raises the blood pressure, which in turn increases stress on the heart.

sodium in salt (Sodium Chloride) that is responsible for the effect on blood pressure. Every gram of salt contains .4 gm of sodium. Or every 1,000 mg of salt contains 400 mg of sodium. (For more details, see page 126)

- **Low Potassium.** The potassium/sodium ratio is of critical importance. Eating more vegetables while reducing salt would greatly increase this ratio and lower elevated blood pressures.
- **Obesity.** Nearly everyone who is significantly overweight will eventually experience high blood pressure. It's usually just a matter of time.
- **Arterial Plaque.** Narrowed and plugged arteries force the body to boost the blood pressure in order to deliver necessary oxygen and food to body cells.

- **Lack of Exercise.**
- **Smoking.**
- **Alcohol.** Scientific studies

> Americans eat more than 10 times the amount of salt their bodies need. And they pay for it with high blood pressure, heart failure, and other problems related to fluid retention.

have demonstrated that even moderate use of alcohol may account for 5 to 15 percent of all hypertension.

Why do Americans eat so much salt?

The most recent guidlines by the American Medical Association suggest a more ideal sodium content of 1,500 mg/day, or less than 5,000 mg of saslt. That is about 5 gm of salt, or one teaspoon of salt. In today's life it's hard to get away from salt. About 75 percent of our salt intake comes from fast and processed foods, and from food eaten in restaurants. A taste for salt is easy to develop, and salty snacks and foods abound to accommodate us.

What about medications for hypertension?

The past few years have produced an avalanche of new drugs that are effective in lowering blood pressure. Some are lifesaving. Most of these drugs produce prompt results—the quick fix that Americans love.

But a closer look at hypertension medications reveals some disquieting facts: the drugs do not cure hypertension; they only control it. Furthermore, these medications have to be taken for life. And they all have side effects, such as fatigue, depression, lack of sexual desire, and impotence. While these drugs help protect against strokes, they do not give much protection against coronary atherosclerosis (the plugging of heart arteries). Some may actually promote atherosclerosis, diabetes, and gouty arthritis.

What are the alternatives?

A number of major scientific studies have shown that simple dietary

WHAT'S YOUR RISK?

	SYSTOLIC	DIASTOLIC
High Blood Pressure *(greater risk of disease)*	130 and above	or 85 and above
	130	85
High Normal BP *(some increased risk of disease)*	120 to 129 or 80 to 84 (high normal)	
	120	80
Optimal Blood Pressure	below 120 and below 80	

Numbers apply to adults who are not taking drugs to lower their blood pressure.

If your systolic and diastolic pressure fall into different categories, your risk depends on the higher category.

Neil Nedley, Proof Positive

Reducing Blood Pressure!

- **Eat lots of fresh, raw foods, both fruits and vegetables. They don't need added salt. They also increase potassium stores, which helps to lower blood pressure.**
- **Look for unsalted snacks (if you need them).**
- **Undercook vegetables and eat them a bit crispy. They will require less salt.**
- **Learn to flavor foods with lemon juice, parsley, tarragon, garlic, or onions, instead of salt.**
- **Lose extra pounds**
- **Reduce the blood viscosity (thin down the blood) by**
  - **reducing fats, oil and grease**
  - **increasing water consumption to 8 to 10 glasses/day.**
- **Increase daily exercise (10,000 steps/day)**
- **Don't smoke or use alcohol.**

Some 62 percent of strokes and 45 percent of heart attacks are related to high blood pressure.

and lifestyle changes can reverse most essential hypertension in a matter of weeks without drugs.

- A large percentage of people are sensitive to salt and would benefit from its reduction in their diets.
- When the weight goes down, blood pressure levels usually fall. Reducing excess weight is often the only treatment needed to correct a rising blood pressure.
- A diet very low in fat yet high in fiber lowers the blood pressure about 10 percent even without weight loss or salt restriction. Thinning of the blood from eating less fat and drinking more water helps produce these benefits.
- Deleting alcohol from the diet will lower blood pressure and will do the body a favor in many other ways.
- Physical exercise lowers blood pressure by reducing peripheral arterial resistance. In addition, regular exercise promotes general health and well-being.

People taking blood pressure medications should not play doctor and change doses or stop medicines on their own. But those who are willing to make healthful lifestyle changes will usually find their physicians glad to help them eat and exercise their way out of hypertension and medication.

NOTES

Every third adult in North America has high blood pressure. This puts them at risk of heart failure, stroke, and other debilitating diseases. Obesity, narrowed arteries, smoking, lack of exercise, estrogen, alcohol, and high salt intake all contribute to the problem. Fortunately, most cases of hypertension can be reversed in weeks by simple dietary and lifestyle changes.

A Tremendous Step

Become a Label Reader

By carefully reading labels, you can select products low in sodium. Watch for such words as "salt," and "sodium," and avoid products in which these terms are listed among the first five ingredients. Reading US nutrition labels, a product is usually "salt-safe," if the number of mg of sodium is not much higher than the number of calories listed per serving

Be aware of the FDA's packaging terminology. Under these guidelines, words appearing on a package have very specific meanings.

FDA'S GUIDELINES

Per Serving	
Sodium-free	under 5 mg
Very Low Sodium	under 35 mg
Low Sodium	under 140 mg
Reduced Sodium	a 75 percent decrease

How About You?

Are you surprised? Does it seem as if just about everything contains enough salt to pickle your insides? Don't despair. By eating an abundance of fresh and unrefined foods, you automatically cut the sodium (and fat) in your diet, and you'll get plenty of protective potassium.

Getting the Salt Out

Not salting your food is a good way to start protecting yourself from stroke. Unfortunately, only some 20 percent of the salt we eat comes from the shaker. Much of the rest is hidden in processed foods and snacks. Here are a few examples:

Some Processed Foods	Salt (mg)
Apple Pie (1 slice)	800
Canned Chili and Beans (1 cup)	3,000
Rice-A-Roni Pilaf (1 cup)	2,500
Wheaties (2 oz)	1,050
Potato Chips (Pringles) (7 oz)	3,000
Tomato Sauce (1/2 cup)	950
Canned Tomato Bisque (1 cup)	1,125
Corned Beef (3 oz)	1,875
Cheese, American (2 slices)	1,350
Kentucky Fried Chicken (3-piece meal)	5,600

NOTES

Stalking a Crippler

"You worry about heart attacks when you pass 50. Strokes, you begin to worry past 60."
—*Don Smith, M.D., Colorado Neurological Institute*

Not only can you survive this grim condition—you can prevent it. Two million Americans lie crippled from paralyzing strokes. After AIDS and cancer, stroke is probably the most dreaded and disabling disease to afflict Westernized civilizations and the third most common cause of death in North America.

What are a person's chances of developing a stroke?

Some 795,000 Americans suffer strokes each year, and 137,000 die from them. As with heart attacks, serious and even fatal strokes can occur without warning. Around one fourth of victims under age 70 die from the first attack; after that the figure doubles.

Of those who survive, 40 percent need some degree of ongoing special care, but only 10 percent require institutionalization.

The remaining 60 percent represent the good news. Some recover completely; nearly all improve enough to care for themselves; most are able to resume their normal activities.

What causes strokes?

A stroke, or cerebral vascular accident (CVA), is most commonly related to atherosclerosis—a thickening, narrowing, and hardening of arteries supplying the brain with oxygenated blood. These atherosclerotic processes can occur both in arteries within the brain and in arteries leading to the brain. The roughened, ragged inner surfaces of damaged arteries become seedbeds for clot formation and plaque buildup. When obstruction is complete, the artery is said to be *thrombosed*.

Sometimes pieces of plaque or blood clots break off from other parts of the circulatory system and travel to smaller brain arteries producing obstruction. These "traveling pieces" are called *emboli*. Some 80 percent of CVAs result from either thrombotic or embolic arterial blockages. Hemorrhages, or blowouts, cause the rest of the strokes. Most of these are associated with uncontrolled high blood

> "Let the morning bring me word of your unfailing love, for I have put my trust in you. Show me the way I should go, for to you I lift up my soul." —Psalm 143:8

pressure that forces blood through cracks in stiffened artery walls. A few blowouts are caused by *aneurysms*, which are ballooned-out areas in arteries that eventually rupture. Either way, the result is bleeding into the brain.

Strokes do their damage by preventing fresh blood from reaching an area of the brain, which soon dies from lack of oxygen. If a large portion of the brain is affected, the stroke will be severe, and can be fatal. A smaller area of brain damage will cause lesser symptoms.

Who is at risk for strokes?

Most strokes are directly related to high blood pressure. People with hypertension are eight times more likely to suffer a stroke than are people with normal blood pressure. Other strokes are related to the presence of atrial fibrillation (irregular heartbeat), which increases the stroke risk six times.

Blackout spells, called *Transient Ischemic Attacks* (TIAs), may be early warnings. These are small strokes that start suddenly and disappear

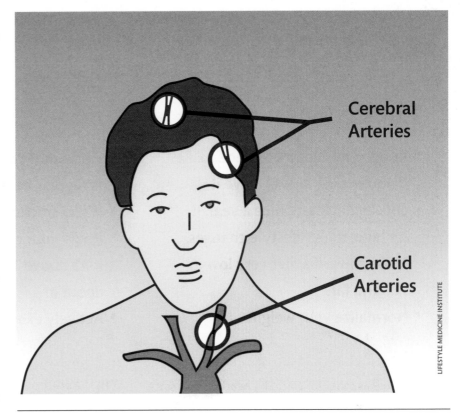

The cerebral and carotid arteries are the most common sites of atherosclerotic plaque buildup associated with strokes.

in less than 24 hours. Most last only a few seconds, and recovery is complete. Persistent TIAs, however, increase the chances for a complete stroke, much as angina attacks increase the chances of a heart attack.

Other risk factors include elevated blood cholesterol and triglycerides, smoking, diabetes, obesity, and sedentary lifestyle. All of these contribute to the atherosclerotic process. In fact, the risk factors for stroke are basi-

In the U.S., stroke is the leading cause of adult disability.

Stroke Warning Signs

Call 9-1-1 immediately if any of the following warning signs appear, since "clotbusters" can neutralize many strokes if given in time:

- Sudden dimness or loss of vision, particularly in one eye.
- Loss of speech, or trouble talking or understanding speech.
- Sudden weakness or numbness of the face, arm, or leg on one side of the body.
- Unexplained dizziness, unsteadiness or sudden falls, especially with any of the above-mentioned symptoms.

Reducing the Risk

- Know your blood pressure. If you're over age 40, have it checked at least twice a year. If it's high, make lifestyle changes. Move toward a diet very low in salt and fat.
- Normalize your weight.

- Find out if you have atrial fibrillation (irregular heart rate).
- If you smoke, stop.
- Know your cholesterol number! If it's above 160 (4.1), then do something about it!
- Actively exercise daily.

cally the same as those for coronary heart disease since both diseases are caused by underlying damage to vital, oxygen-carrying arteries.

Can strokes be prevented?

Yes, most strokes can be prevented. In fact, strokes, like certain other lifestyle diseases, could become relatively uncommon within a generation if people would begin adopting, early in life, the healthful lifestyle practices already known today. These include the following:

- ☐ Don't smoke. One out of every six CVA deaths is directly related to tobacco use.
- ☐ Check blood pressure regularly. Hypertension has no symptoms, and it can sneak up on the unaware.
- ☐ Learn to use much less salt. In areas of the world where salt intake is low, hypertension is virtually unknown. In Japan, where salt intake was high, stroke was the leading cause of death.
- ☐ Normalize weight. Obesity promotes atherosclerosis, hypertension, and diabetes.
- ☐ Eat a diet very low in fat and cholesterol, yet high in fiber. Experiments have shown that keeping fat below 15 percent and cholesterol as low as possible protects the arterial linings from the artery-narrowing atherosclerosis.
- ☐ Exercise actively and regularly. Exercise improves circulation and helps control weight and hypertension.

What about people who have already had strokes? Is there help for them?

Definitely. The lifestyle that helps prevent strokes will also hasten recovery, as well as help prevent recurrent strokes.

Acute strokes require good nursing care and energetic rehabilitation involving intensive and consistent physical therapy.

Small doses of aspirin have been shown to help prevent some strokes in susceptible people, especially people with atrial fibrillation. Remember, however, that aspirin may also promote bleeding tendencies (hemorrhagic strokes) and aggravate stomach ulcers.

The best news, however, is that arterial narrowing is reversible. Thickened, narrowed arteries slowly open again when a very-low-fat vegetarian diet is consistently followed, along with the other health practices. While these studies, so far, center on coronary arteries, similar results are expected in arteries affecting the brain, since the underlying problem is basically the same.

Everyone is born with soft, flexible, elastic artery walls. Many populations around the world retain their healthy arteries and low blood pressures throughout their life. We can, too, if we get serious about pursuing healthful lifestyle practices before the damage occurs.

Stroke is one of the most dreaded and disabling diseases, but it is not a disease that attacks indiscriminately. In many populations around the world, stroke is virtually unknown. You can reduce your risk by adopting a lifestyle that promotes healthy arteries and low blood pressure.

Change Your Bad Habits to Good

Getting the Salt Out

Most of us need to reduce our salt intake. Don't worry about not getting enough salt. If you are like most Americans, you eat more than 10 times the amount the body needs. Three main contributors to this salt excess are:

• Table Salt

Don't add salt at the table. You probably get too much already from the food you eat. Don't add to the problem by pouring more on. Your food will seem bland for a few weeks, but your taste buds will soon adjust, and you will begin to enjoy the subtle flavors of foods. The day will come when foods you now think of as delicious will taste salty.

• Salty Snacks

Things like potato chips, pretzels, and salted nuts are so dangerous they should have a warning from the Surgeon General on the box: "Warning: salty snacks are linked to hypertension, stroke, and heart disease. Eat at your own risk." If you must snack, use substitutes like carrot sticks and sliced apples.

• Fast Foods

Cutting salt intake to less than five grams a day (one teaspoonful) may reduce (if not eliminate) high blood pressure. But you will never reach that goal until you break the fast-food habit. A Hardee's Monster Thickburger alone cotains seven (7) grams of salt. And Arby's Breakfast Sausage Biscuit has more than nine (9) grams of salt. And that bag of "regular" French Fries from Dairy Queen has almost 4 gm of salt. So, beware of fast foods!!

Substitute

Get yourself started in a new direction. Use salt-free spice blends, such as *Mrs. Dash*, to liven up your food.

How About You?

List several things you can do to reduce your risk of stroke:

_____

_____

_____

_____

_____

_____

_____

_____

_____

_____

_____

_____

_____

Do-it-yourself Cancers

Many cancers are turning out to be do-it-yourself diseases. We promote them by chronic exposure to certain environmental factors. What we eat and drink, where we live and work, and what we breathe may well determine whether we become a cancer statistic.

Are you saying that people can bring on their own cancers?

Medical science continues to make strides toward earlier detection and improved treatments for many cancers. But these efforts are largely after the fact. The sad truth is that the overall death rates for many adult cancers have actually gone up. Cancer now claims one in four American lives. It's becoming increasingly obvious: what we eat and drink, where we live and work, and what we breathe can greatly influence whether or not we get cancer.

We can reverse the trend. How? By simply taking the precautions that we already know about. This would probably prevent 70 to 80 percent of the cancers that afflict Americans today.

Won't people do just about anything to avoid such a terrifying disease?

They would do almost anything, it seems, except change their lifestyles.

Take lung cancer (the cancer that kills more men and women in the United States than any other), for example. Ever since the Surgeon General's report in 1964, we've known that lung cancer is directly related to Tabacco smoking. It's true that millions have quit smoking, yet every fourth adult in North America

DEATHS FROM SMOKING/YEAR

Lung cancer	125,500
All other cancers	35,500
Cardiovascular disease	129,000
Respiratory diseases	103,000
Smoking-related fires	1,500
Babies because of smoking mothers	2,000
Passive smoking	46,500
TOTAL FROM SMOKING	**443,000**

> "Test everything. Hold on to the good. Avoid every kind of evil."
> —1 Thessalonians 5:21, 22

still smokes! In addition, some 90 percent of the cancers of the lung, lip, mouth, tongue, throat, and esophagus could be prevented if people simply stopped using tobacco. And it would also prevent half the bladder cancers.

Are some cancers related to diet?

In men, the second and third most frequently occurring cancers are those of the prostate and colon. For women it's cancers of the breast and colon. Extensive evidence links nearly 50 percent of these cancers to overnutrition—too much fat, too much aniaml protein and too much weight.

That sounds like a long shot. Wouldn't a more likely culprit be the many chemicals that find their way into our food supply?

Carcinogens (cancer-producing chemicals) are a concern—especially with the array of additives, preservatives, flavor enhancers, pesticides, and other chemicals that we use in producing and marketing food. However, only 2 percent of all cancers can be reliably linked to these substances.

In contrast, evidence of the connection between cancer and such dietary factors as fiber, animal protein and fat grows stronger every day. Compared with diets around 1900, the average American now eats one third more fat, twice as much animal protein and one third less fiber (see page 122). In areas of the world in which fat and animal protein intake is low and fiber consumption is high, the incidence of colon, breast, and prostate cancers are negligible. In countries, such as the United States, Canada, Australia, and New Zealand, where diets are low in fiber and high in fat, and animal protein, the rates for these kinds of cancers are much higher.

Could ethnic variations, rather than diet, account for these differences?

Researchers asked the same question. In a study published in 1979, they found, for example, that Japanese living in Japan had very few of these cancers. In Japan, fiber consumption then was high and fat and animal protein intake low (less than 15 percent of total calories). But when these Japanese migrated to Hawaii and adopted Western eating habits

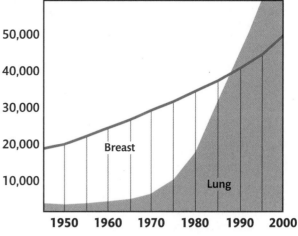

CANCER DEATH TRENDS FOR U.S. WOMEN

and lifestyles, their rates for these cancers increased dramatically and soon equaled those for other Americans.

How can such things as dietary fat, animal protein and fiber affect cancer rates?

Not all the answers are in yet, but cancer is associated with carcinogens—chemical irritants that can produce cancerous lesions over time.

Bile acids are an example. The amount of fat in the diet affects the amount of bile the body produces. In the intestinal tract some of these bile acids can form irritating carcinogenic compounds. The longer these compounds stay in contact with the lining of the colon, the more irritation results.

Breast Cancer Trends

1960 = 1 in 20

1980 = 1 in 11

2000 = 1 in 7

CANCER MORTALITY RISK DIFFERENTIAL OF JAPANESE IMMIGRANTS

Cancer	Japanese		Caucasians in Hawaii
	in Japan	in Hawaii	
Breast	1x	4x	6x
Colon	1x	5x	5x
Prostate	1x	11x	3x
Rectum	1x	3x	2x
Lung	1x	2x	4x

Nitrites are another example. Nitrites are used to preserve processed meat and to give cured meats their recognizable color. These can form N-nitroso compounds involved in carcinogenesis.

This is where fiber comes in. With a low-fiber diet, digested food moves slowly through the intestines, often taking from three to five days to complete the journey from entry to exit. Interestingly enough, most fibers absorb water like a sponge. This helps fill the intestines and stimulates them to increased activity. The high fiber content speeds up the transit time, and food now travels through the intestines in 24 to 36 hours.

This helps the colon in two ways. It shortens the exposure time to irritating substances, and it dilutes the concentration of the carcinogens as they pass through the colon thanks to fiber's water-holding ability and insulating effect.

PERCENT OF FATAL CANCERS RELATED TO ALCOHOL

	Percentage
Esophagus	75
Mouth	50
Larynx	50
Breast	40
Liver	30

Most Cancer Is Preventable

How does diet relate to breast and prostate cancers?

A high fat intake depresses the activity of important cells in the body's immune system. This effect has been studied extensively in connection with breast cancer and may affect other types of cancer as well. Dairy products, while possibly being protective for colon cancer, have been clearly implicated in raising the risk for prostate cancer.

Are other lifestyle areas connected to cancer?

Alcohol consumption increases the risk for cancer of the esophagus, breast, liver, and colon, and does so dramatically for those who smoke as well. Excess weight raises the risk of cancer of the breast, colon, endometrium, kidney, pancreas and gallbladder. Then there are such things as exposure to asbestos, sidestream smoke, and toxic chemicals.

Summary

Surprisingly, just four lifestyle factors could prevent close to 80 percent of the adult cancers found in Westernized society today: (1) no smoking, (2) no alcohol, (3) a vegetarian diet that's very low in fat and high in fiber, and (4) normal weight. Instead of one American in four dying of cancer, the risk could be reduced to one in 20.

It's not an impossible dream.

The Risks of Cancer

Tobacco	Smoking causes one of every three cancer deaths in North America.
Red Meat	Regular meat eaters have a three times higher risk of developing colon cancer when compared with occasional meat eaters.
Junk Food	Those who fill up on doughnuts, sodas, and potato chips lose out on the cancer-fighting substances found in fruits and vegetables.
Inactivity	Those who log at least four hours of exercise a week cut their risk of breast and colon cancer by more than a third.
Overeating	Among women, being heavy adds markedly to the danger from breast, colon, and endometrial cancer. And men are pushing their luck with pancreatic and colon cancers.
Alcohol	Excessive drinking has been clearly linked to cancers of the liver, throat, colon and esophagus. In women, even a daily drink or two raises the breast cancer risk.
Dairy	Diets high in calcium and dairy are linked with increased prostate cancer risk.

Lifestyle factors, such as smoking, obesity, consumption of alcohol, and a diet high in animal products and fat, account for up to 80 percent of all cancers.

Miracle Cure?

Imagine the announcement of a pill that would make people immune to cancer. It would be the news story of the decade. People would flock to their doctors for a prescription, and the inventors would be wealthy beyond belief.

No such pill exists. But there are a number of things we can do for ourselves to prevent the majority of adult cancers.

A good place to start is with our food. We can begin eating a diet considerably lower in fat and cholesterol. Many studies have shown that such a diet reduces the risk of heart disease, diabetes, stroke, and many types of cancer.

But making lifestyle changes is not as simple as swallowing a pill. It involves learning new habits and skills. For example, cutting the fat and cholesterol in our diet means preparing more meatless dishes.

One sensible way to develop these skills is by designating a day or two each week for vegetarian-style meals. This gives you a chance to experiment with healthful ways of cooking while gradually building up a new repertoire of favorite new recipes.

Good Eating Begins With Good Recipes

A good cookbook is an investment that will repay you many times over. There's no better tool when it comes to changing your eating habits. (See Educational Resources, pp. 253-256.)

Lifesaving Tests

Beat cancer by detecting it early. The odds of surviving colon cancer are nine in 10 when it's discovered before it spreads, but only one in 14 afterward.

What's more, a full 97 percent of women diagnosed with localized breast cancer are alive five years later, compared to only 20 percent of those found to have metastasized breast cancer.

Breast
- **Self-examination** monthly from age 20. Any new or suspicious lumps should be checked by a doctor.
- **Breast exam** every three years from age 20 to 39, then annually.
- **Mammogram** every year or two from age 40.

Cervix
- **Pelvic exam** with Pap smear annually from age 18 and for younger women who are sexually active. After three consecutive normal results, some doctors recommend testing less frequently.

Skin
- Self-examination once a month. Look for unusual pearly bumps or red scaly patches. Also check for moles that have changed size or color, or have begun to ooze or bleed easily.

Colon
- Fecal occult blood test annually after age 50.
- Digital rectal exam, performed as part of a standard physical exam, annually after age 40.
- Colonoscopy, an exam of the large intestine every 10 years after age 50.

Prostate
- Prostate-specific antigen (PSA) test annually after age 50.
- Digital rectal exam, as part of a standard physical exam, annually after age 40.

MOVING TOWARD *THE OPTIMAL DIET*

- **Use whole-grain breads and cereals.** They have the vitamins, minerals, and fiber that refined flour products don't have.
- **Enjoy a variety of fresh fruit each day.**
- **Eat a wide variety of vegetables.** Dark-green leafy vegetables are essential for good health! For instance, one cup of greens may contain more calcium than milk. And yellow and orange vegetables are high in vitamin A.
- **Enjoy nuts.** They are high in minerals and vitamins, but use them sparingly because they are high in fat and calories.
- **Use a wide variety of beans and peas.** They provide protein and fiber, and they are low in fat.

Disarming Diabetes

In America every third person has either pre-diabetes or full-blown diabetes.

S ince World War II diabetes has been advancing relentlessly. It has now become one of the leading causes of death. In North America, babies born today will have a one in three chance of developing diabetes in their lifetime. Until recent times, there has been no known cure.

And yet, many people are now actually beating diabetes. They are normalizing their blood sugars, and they are getting off insulin. They do this by making better lifestyle choices.

What exactly is diabetes?

Diabetes occurs when the body becomes unable to handle glucose (sugar), which builds up to dangerous levels in the blood. A diagnosis of diabetes is usually made when a blood sugar test is consistently above 125 mg% (7.0 mmol/L) after an eight-hour fast. Fasting blood sugar (FBS) levels of 100-125 (5.6-6.9 mmol/L) are known as prediabetes.

There are two kinds of diabetes. Type I afflicts about 5 percent of diabetics. They are usually thin and have a defective pancreatic issue that no longer produces sufficient, if any, insulin. This type of diabetes usually begins in childhood and is commonly known as juvenile diabetes. Since these diabetics cannot survive without insulin, it is now officially called insulin-dependent diabetes mellitus (IDDM).

Type II diabetes is different. Called adult-onset diabetes, or noninsulin-dependent diabetes mellitus (NIDDM), it is the most common kind, affecting more than 90 percent of diabetics. While this type generally hits around age 50 as people get older and fatter, some people with the recent epidemic of obesity are developing this disease now in their teens. In contrast to the juvenile diabetics, most Type II diabetics have plenty of insulin in their bodies when diagnosed, but something diminishes the insulin's ability to do its job effectively.

There is only one body per customer. It's entrusted to you. Treat it with respect!

In America every third person has either pre-diabetes or full-blown diabetes.

What are the warning signs of diabetes?

The classical symptoms are polydipsia (excessive thirst), polyphagia (excessive appetite), and polyuria (excessive passage of urine). Early in the disease, however, few symptoms show up—perhaps some increase in urinary frequency and thirst. Of the 25.8 million diabetics in America it is estimated that 7 million don't even know that they have it. With another 79 million being in the pre-diabetic category, some 104 million Americans are at risk. That's every third man, woman, and child! As the disease progresses, its effects are devastating affecting all organs of the body and gradually destroying them. Consider the risks of unrecognized or poorly controlled diabetes:

- Eight out of 10 diabetics develop eye problems. Diabetes is the leading cause of new blindness in developed countries.
- Diabetics are 18 times more likely to experience serious kidney damage than are nondiabetics. Some 25 percent of kidney dialysis patients are diabetics.
- Diabetes is a potent promoter of atherosclerosis (narrowing and hardening of the arteries). The result is that diabetes more than doubles the risk of heart attacks and strokes. It can also lead to sexual impotence, hearing impairment, intermittent claudication (disabling leg cramps) and gangrene (half of all foot and leg

amputations in adults are from this cause).

What causes Type II diabetes?

Studies demonstrate a strong

Walk Away From Diabetes

relationship to fat—both fat in the diet and fat on the body. The disease is not as common in areas of the world where fat intake and obesity rates are low.

Normally insulin, a pancreatic hormone, enables body cells to use glucose and controls blood sugar levels. But most of the time the problem in Type II diabetes is not a defective pancreas unable to produce sufficient insulin, but a lack of sensitivity to insulin. This resistance of the cells to insulin appears to relate directly to obesity and to excess fat in the diet and possibly in the liver.

But isn't sugar the culprit?

James Anderson, M.D., professor of medicine and clinical nutrition at the College of Medicine, University of Kentucky, and a widely respected authority on diabetes, evaluated the effect of diet on blood sugar levels. Just as others had done before him, Dr. Anderson was able to turn lean healthy young men into mild diabetics in less than two weeks by feeding them a rich 65 percent fat diet. A similar group, fed a lean 10 percent fat diet plus one pound of sugar a day, did not produce even

one diabetic after 11 weeks when the experiment was terminated.

So what's the best way to treat this disease?

Several treatment centers have convincingly demonstrated that most Type II diabetics can normalize their blood sugar levels, often `within weeks, by following a simple plant food-centered diet, very low in fat and high in fiber, coupled with daily exercise.

Lowering the amount of fat, oil, and grease in the diet plays the crucial role. When less fat is eaten, less fat reaches the bloodstream and the liver. This begins a complicated process that gradually restores the sensitivity to insulin, which can then facilitate the entry of sugar from the bloodstream into the body cells. The effect is often dramatic. A Type II diabetic who lowers daily fat intake to about 10 percent of total calories can often normalize the blood sugar levels within weeks. Many are eventually able to get off diabetic medication entirely—both pills and injections.

Eating more natural, fiber-rich foods plays an important role by helping stabilize blood sugar levels. When foods are eaten without their normal complement of fiber, blood sugar levels can quickly shoot up. Normally a surge of insulin then counteracts this. People who consume refined foods, drinks, and snacks high in calories but low in fiber may experience hikes and dips in blood sugar levels all day long. High-fiber foods, on the other hand,

Start now. Beat diabetes before it happens.

A STUDY confirms that even small amounts of weight gain can increase your risk of developing Type II diabetes, according to the American Journal of Epidemiology. A five-pound gain increases your risk for diabetes by 10 percent.

The earlier that diabetes is detected, the more likely lifestyle modifications are going to be effective.

It's your future. Be there!

DIABETES TRENDS BY AGE GROUP

% diabetics

The National Diabetes Data Group (NIH)

65-74 years

55-64 years

45-54 years

The percentage of diabetics for selected age groups has steadily increased; i.e., the diabetes rate for those 45 to 54 years has gone from 1 in 1950 to 10 in 2005, an increase of 1,000 percent (or %). (U.S. 1950-2005)

smooth out these blood sugar fluctuations and stabilize energy levels.

Active physical exercise has an insulin-like reaction in that it burns up the excess fuel (blood sugar and fatty acids) more rapidly.

The foremost recommended lifestyle modification for diabetes, however, is losing excess weight. Obesity is far and away the most common non-genetic component contributing to the development of diabetes.

Normalizing body weight is often all that is necessary to bring the blood sugar back to normal. The low-fat, high-fiber diet will greatly aid this effort, as will regular, active exercise.

What about Type I diabetes?

Insulin-dependent, or Type I, diabetics will need to take insulin for life until pancreatic transplants become feasible and affordable. However, the high-fiber, very-low-fat diet will help reduce the amount of insulin required to maintain stable blood sugar levels and reduce the ever-present threat of vascular complications.

A protein has been identified in cow's milk that can increase the risk of diabetes in babies. This is one of of the reasons why the American Academy of

Pediatrics recommends that cow's milk should NOT be given to babies until they are at least 1 year of age. Breast-fed infants have been found with a significant measure of protection against this kind of diabetes.

The Outlook

The earlier the detection of diabetes, the more likely lifestyle modifications will be effective. Earlier detection thus takes much of the emphasis off drugs and insulin injections; both of these are costly and come with undesirable side effects.

Remember: the very lifestyle measures that can disarm and normalize many cases of Type II diabetes can also prevent this disease in the first place. Even losing as little as 10 extra pounds and taking a brisk walk a few times a week can help stave off the disease.

Application

One in three people in North America develop diabetes at some point in their life, yet this disease can be prevented and sometimes even cured. The secret? Low fat, both in the diet and on the body.

Low-Fat Checklist

The main villain in Type II diabetes is the enormous amount of fat in our diet. One way we can reduce this overabundance is by using less fat, oil, and grease during cooking. How many of the following do you do?

Use non-stick (teflon) cookware to minimize the amount of oil needed to keep food from sticking.

_____ Cook onions, green peppers, and other vegetables in broth instead of browning in fat.

_____ Use less oil, butter, or fat than a recipe calls for.

_____ Eliminate the dabs of butter from casserole toppings and vegetables.

_____ Use a non-stick spray or a film of lecithin instead of greasing a casserole dish.

_____ Avoid frying.

_____ Cook only very lean meat (or better yet, eat no meat at all).

_____ Steam or microwave vegetables instead of sautéeing them in butter or oil.

What can you do?

What steps can you take to reduce the fat in your diet?

_____

_____

_____

_____

_____

_____

_____

How to Beat Diabetes (Type II)

Diabetes is a leading cause of new blindness, foot and leg amputations, and hearing impairment. The worst part is that many people suffer needlessly. Here is the formula that can help beat this disease.

1. Eat more natural fiber-rich foods, simply prepared, low in fat, grease, and sugar. Freely use whole-grain products, tubers and legumes, salads and vegetables. Eat a substantial breakfast daily—a hot multigrain cereal will curb your appetite for hours and stabilize your blood sugar.

2. As a diabetic, use fresh whole fruits, but not more than three servings a day. Don't use fruit juices.

3. Avoid refined and processed foods. They are usually high in fat and sugar, and low in fiber.

4. Markedly reduce fats, oils, and grease. If you use animal products, use them lean and very sparingly, more like a condiment. And avoid oily and creamy dressings and sauces.

5. Walk briskly each day. Two 30-minute walks every day are ideal to help burn up the extra sugar in your blood.

6. Regularly see a physician experienced in the effects of dietary therapy to monitor and adjust your medication needs.

Building Better Bones

Protein is an essential component of a healthy diet. But when we eat too much of it—especially animal protein—then it can be harmful.

Has ordinary, everyday calcium turned out to be the gallant gladiator that can deliver fair maidens from brittle bones, fractured hips, and deformed spines? That is what the calcium manufacturers and the dairy industry would like us to believe. In reality, osteoporosis is far more complicated than that.

What is osteoporosis?

Osteoporosis (literally, porous bone) silently and painlessly weakens the bones of 25 million Americans. Previously sturdy bones gradually become thin and fragile, their interiors soft and spongy. As a result, bones break, giving rise to the term *brittle bones*.

Osteoporosis may cause as many as 1.3 million fractures a year. Hip fractures can be both disabling and deadly. Spinal fractures, on the other hand, are often painless, but can rob a person of two to eight inches of height. The resultant spinal curvature is the source of dowager's hump.

How does osteoporosis develop?

Normal bones continue to increase in strength and thickness until around age 35. Then the process gradually reverses itself, and small amounts of bone density is being lost each year. This loss accelerates in women after menopause and can continue for seven to 15 years. When risk factors are present, bone loss occurs even faster, and osteoporosis may develop.

Although usually considered a disease of older women, 20 percent of victims are men.

How can I tell if I have it?

Without professional help, you can't—not until you fracture a bone or start shrinking in height, and that's quite late in the disease. Earlier diagnosis is best done by physicians at reliable medical centers.

If you are middle-aged or older and you have two or more of the following risk factors, you should be tested:

* sedentary lifestyle
* early menopause
* chronic use of corticosteroids
* cigarettes, caffeine, or alcohol use
* standard American diet high in animal protein, and salt.

What can be done to treat this disease?

Several treatments are being used:

Estrogen therapy. When used, it slows down bone loss, but increases the risk for uterine and breast cancer, thrombophlebitis (blood clots) and gallbladder disease. It may also aggravate diabetes and hypertension, and women sometimes face periodic uterine biopsies. Over the years, adding progesterone was designed to blunt some of these disturbing side effects. The results of the large Women's Health Initiative, however, have raised so much concern about the use of these hormones that many physicians prescribe them now only for special clinical conditions, such as severe hot flashes, and even then, only for a short time.

Vitamin D. The body uses vitamin D to absorb calcium, but most Americans get more than they need if they have sufficient sun exposure. A 15-minute face-to-the-sun exposure may give you a jolt of 20,000 IU of vitamin D! The dietary recommendations is 600 to 800 IU/day.

Calcium. Various U.S. governmental agencies have recommended 1,200 to 1,500 milligrams of calcium a day. Until recently, the World Health Organization (WHO), however, recommended only 500 mg since calcium deficiency has never been documented anywhere in the world, even with calcium intakes of as little as 300 milligrams a day. With westernization of most diets, and the increase in osteoporosis, the WHO is now recommending 1,000 mg of calcium/day (see table next page).

Exercise. Bones will not thicken and strengthen without regular, weight-bearing exercise, such as walking. To retain their minerals, bones need to be pressed, pushed, pulled, and twisted against gravity.

The gravity factor was well demonstrated by the early astronauts. Even though they exercised faithfully while in space, their bones showed startling osteoporotic changes on their return. While nearly all types of aerobic exercise are beneficial to the body, what the bones need most is a good daily shake-up.

- **If you smoke, stop!** It will do your bones a big favor.
- **Reduce the amount of animal protein, salt, and caffeine in the diet.** Osteoporosis appears to be a disease of affluence and *excess*, rather than one of *deficiency*. Osteoporosis is a rather complex disease largely related to our dietary lifestyle. The standard American diet, high in animal protein, salt, phosphorus (meat, certain soft drinks), and caffeine, causes calcium to be leached from the bones and excreted in the urine. These lifestyle-induced calcium losses seem to override any amount of calcium consumed or swallowed.

What's the evidence for this connection?

Eskimos consume diets extremely high in both protein (250 to 400 grams/day) and calcium (1,500 to 2,500 mg/day). In spite of their high calcium intake and the very active lives they lead, they have one of the highest rates of osteoporosis in the world.

The Bantu tribes in Africa, on the other hand, consume an average of 47 gm of protein and less than 400 mg of calcium a day, predominantly from plant foods. Yet, even though Bantu women bear an average of 10 children, which makes special demands on calcium reserves, they are essentially free of osteoporosis. In contrast, relatives of the Bantu who

HOW EASY IT IS TO EAT TOO MUCH PROTEIN!

		Protein (gm)
Breakfast	3-egg ham and cheese omelette	46
	Hash brown potatoes	3
	Toast (2) with butter and jelly	5
	Coffee with cream	1
	Orange juice	1
Lunch	Big Mac	26
	French fries	3
	Milk shake	11
Dinner	Fried chicken	55
	Peas	5
	Mixed salad with dressing	4
	Baked potato with sour cream	9
	Milk (2%), 1 glass	9
	Total	**178 gm**
	Recommended	**50 gm**

Use It or Lose It

In its efficiency the body deposits minerals when there is extra demand placed upon the bones. Exercise stresses bone structure, producing small electrical charges that cause calcium and other minerals to be drawn in and held. "Use it or lose it" is an adage that certainly applies to keeping bones strong.

Vegetarians have an advantage in that their diet is more alkaline, a condition that favors bone density. Part of the body's response to excess acid-forming foods like animal protein and phosphorus-containing foods is to release calcium from the bones."What we need is not more calcium intake, but less calcium loss!"

have migrated to South Africa or the United States and adopted the richer Western dietary lifestyle eventually experience a rate of osteoporosis comparable to that of the rest of the host country's population.

How about prevention?

Many populations around the world average less than 500 mg of calcium a day without any evidence of osteoporosis. It's strangely paradoxical that osteoporosis has become epidemic in the United States, where the consumption of calcium-rich dairy products and calcium supplements is the highest in the world.

DAILY CALCIUM RECOMMENDATIONS

	RDA
U.S. National Academy of Sciences	**1,200 mg**
U.S. National Institute of Health (for post-menopausal women to combat the osteoporosis epidemic in North America)	**1,500 mg**
World Health Organization (In developing countries with daily calcium intake usually at 300-500 mg, osteoporosis is rarely found.	**1,000 mg**

Most Americans eat twice as much protein than they need (see pages 102-105). Reducing protein intake to the Recommended Daily Intake (RDI) of 50 to 60 grams a day, along with daily active exercise and a healthful diet low in salt, phosphorus, and caffeine, holds promise of turning the tide in the battle against brittle bones.

NOTES

Application

Osteoporosis is epidemic in North America, even though the consumption of calcium-rich dairy products and supplements is the highest in the world. By reducing the intake of animal protein, salt, caffeine, and phosphorus, and by adopting a program of daily exercise, we can turn the tide in the battle against this crippling disease.

The Case of the Unsuccessful Savers

Janice and Steve have trouble saving money. Once the bills are paid, nothing ever seems to be left. After some serious discussion, Janice decided to take a part-time job, and Steve asked his boss for more overtime hours.

What a difference! The next month their paychecks were larger than ever before. But once again, no money was left once the bills had been paid. Janice and Steve had increased their spending to match their new income.

Spending Calcium

Something similar happens to people eating a diet high in animal protein and salt. The body "spends" calcium as it processes animal protein, salt, and caffeine. When there is not enough calcium available in the diet, it "borrows" from another source—the bones and teeth!

The Western diet provides two times the recommended daily allowance of protein. At the same time, it provides 10 times more salt than the body requires. At this level it is almost impossible to get enough calcium to balance the losses. Slowly over the years the bones become brittle and weak.

The solution is not to take more calcium, but to eat less animal protein, salt, and caffeine. This allows the body to conserve the calcium already stored in the bones.

High-Calcium, High-Protein Foods

Chart 1 lists some typical sources of calcium. Notice how high they are in animal protein. With some of these foods you get a lot of calcium, but you may lose even more as the body has to deal with the excess animal protein.

High-Calcium, Low-Protein Foods

Chart 2 also lists good sources of calcium. But this time, note the moderate amounts of protein—and coming from plant sources—provided by these foods. Another bonus is that they are all low in fat and cholesterol-free.

1. CALCIUM IN CONCENTRATED PROTEIN FOODS

	Serving Size	Calcium (in mg)	Protein (in gm)
Beef, Chicken	5 ounces	15	34-45
Cheddar cheese	4 slices	900	35
Whole milk	3 glasses	875	27

2. CALCIUM IN UNCONCENTRATED PROTEIN FOODS

	Serving Size	Calcium (in mg)	Protein (in gm)
Collard greens	1 cup	360	5
Spinach, Broccoli	1 cup	175	5
Bread	2 slices	50-90	5

Save More Than You Spend

Everyone knows that you can't save money when you spend more than you make. The same principle applies to calcium: You can't keep bones strong if you're flushing the calcium out of them with a diet high in animal protein, salt, excessive caffeine and phosphorus.

How Tough Are Your Bones?

Try to cut down on calcium-robbing, high-protein meats and dairy products. Instead, look to lower protein sources of calcium found in whole grains, dark-green leafy vegetables, and beans.

Disease With a Thousand "Cures"

"At age 89 it's a wonderful thing to get up in the morning and not hurt anywhere."
—Mavis Lindgren, marathon runner

B ecause arthritis is a chronic disease that never quite seems to go away, even with good medical treatment, hundreds of folk remedies have grown up around it. And there are hundreds more unproven, expensive, and often outright quack treatments being offered to vulnerable arthritis sufferers by unscrupulous promoters.

How would you define arthritis?

Arthritis is a general term for diseases or other abnormal processes occurring in the joints. An estimated 40 million Americans suffer from some form of arthritis.

Our joints and ligaments, like our muscles, wear with use and need to be constantly repaired—a process that normally occurs during sleep. Repair of any body part requires free access to oxygen and other nutrients. When circulation of the blood becomes inadequate, ligaments weaken, joint fluids decrease, and cartilage wears away.

What is the most common form of arthritis?

Osteoarthritis is the most common type, and is almost universally present in older populations. It can also occur at any time after an injury (called traumatic arthritis) or with excessive wear and tear to a joint, as often happens in football.

Osteoarthritis usually occurs when a joint's blood supply becomes inadequate for its needed function. Just as a heart will weaken and ultimately fail when the coronary arteries clog up with plaque, so joints begin to break down when the arteries supplying them become narrowed or obstructed. For this reason most osteoarthritis responds to measures that improve circulation, such

"Pleasant words are a honeycomb, sweet to the soul and healing to the bones." —Proverbs 16:24

as lowering the amount of fat in the bloodstream, regular exercise, and hydrotherapy (water treatments).

Osteoarthritis of weight-bearing joints, such as the spine, knees, and hips, is commonly aggravated by caloric overload (obesity). Just as a bridge has a load limit, so do the joints.

The most common symptoms of osteoarthritis are pain and stiffness, which tend to decrease as the joint is warmed up with activity.

Are backaches caused by arthritis?

Backaches afflict more than 5 million Americans every year—four out of five people will suffer from them at some time in their lives. Back problems are important because they are a leading cause of disability, missed workdays, and many lawsuits.

Surprisingly, up to 80 percent of low back sufferers are victims of overworked or underexercised muscles. A strained muscle may suddenly go into a sustained contraction or spasm and become a hard knotty mass, signaling body distress by sharp pain.

Another 10 percent of back problems may be caused by osteoarthritis or a disc problem. Only a very few who suffer from back pain have a specific serious injury.

When a backache occurs, it's important to rule out an identifiable injury before anything else is done. Without an evident serious problem, the important thing is not to do what you feel like—retiring to a soft sofa. Keep the rest to one day after injury or onset of pain, or two at the most.

At this stage ice bags are helpful, along with doctor-prescribed muscle relaxants and nonsteroidal anti-inflammatory medications.

Then it's time to get up on your feet and start walking. Walk through the pain. Back specialists say that prolonged bed rest will do more harm than good, because rest causes

How does a joint tell you it's not getting enough blood? It usually begins to hurt!

your back muscles to weaken rapidly. Instead of becoming reconditioned, you become deconditioned. After a while even light activity may sprain or strain muscles barely able to carry their own weight.

Fortunately most back problems resolve themselves in four to 12 weeks. Here are a few tips to prevent recurrence, or to prevent backaches entirely.

- Keep your weight down—the biggest favor you can do for your back.
- Avoid high heels (over one inch). They tilt the pelvis and throw the back out of alignment.
- Strengthen your back and abdominal muscles with special exercises. Walk, swim, or jog at least 20 minutes five times a week.
- Eat a diet very low in fat and high in fiber to improve your circulation, better allowing

the blood to carry extra oxygen and nutrients to the compromised areas.

These measures are important for all kinds of arthritis as well as for back pain.

What about the painful, swollen big toe?

You mean gout, or gouty arthritis. From antiquity this disease has been associated with the lifestyle of the rich: too many rich foods and too little exercise. You can still see pictures in old history books of such kings, with a foot propped up on a footstool, protecting that painful big toe.

Sometimes the afflicted royal person was sent to live and work with the peasants. This was effective because the simpler diet and a more active life eventually reversed the disease.

We now know that some metabolic weakness may be involved in gout. But we also know that it can be controlled by simplifying the diet and by eliminating the offending purines (largely from the breakdown of animal protein) and normalizing weight.

What about red swollen joints?

You are probably thinking of rheumatoid arthritis. This is different from osteoarthritis in that it results from inflammation of the joints with redness, swelling, pain, and fever, rather than from injury or wear and tear.

Rheumatoid arthritis is an autoimmune disease, related to asthma, hay fever, eczema, and other diseases that have an allergic component. Acute attacks tend to recur

The surprising answer to arthritis pain? Exercise!

Since cartilage (the pad between the bones) doesn't have a blood supply, it has to get its nutrients from the joint lining, which occurs only when the joint is used.

over the years, producing nodules and gradually stiffening and disfiguring the joints, most notably the wrist and finger joints.

Rheumatoid arthritis has long been known to be closely intertwined with the body's immune (defense) system. Certain immune protein complexes deposited in the joints play a key role in the marked destruction of cartilage that takes place. We now know that these undesirable protein antigens (perpetrators of allergies) can be absorbed intact from the small intestine without being digested, thus causing the problems.

Dietary habits are believed important because studies of rural populations in developing countries show a fraction of the incidence of rheumatoid arthritis that is found among their urban counterparts. Other studies have demonstrated that when eating foods associated with few allergic symptoms, patients experience less stiffness and pain, and improvement in muscle strength. In addition, any lifestyle measures designed to improve circulation are important as well.

The best long-term results are seen in patients willing to adopt a very strict vegan diet (without any animal products). This is not surprising, since milk is the most common cause of food allergies, with eggs close behind. Studies have shown, for example, that more than 100 antigens may be released during the digestion of cow's milk alone.

Fight for your health. Stay active. The people who get better are the ones who take an active role in bringing about positive, permanent changes in their lifestyles.

NOTES

Healing Moves
for Aching Joints

Can you summarize some practical guidelines for preventing or reversing the effects of chronic arthritis?

Despite the many different forms of arthritis, here are some general principles that are effective in most cases:

1. Normalize your weight. Every extra pound increases the wear and tear of the main weight-bearing joints—the hips, knees, and spine.

2. Simplify your diet. Diets very low in fat and high in fiber have been shown to improve circulation to the joints. In time, this kind of diet may help open up some of the narrowed arteries. Eliminate all dairy products for three weeks and evaluate your response.

3. Exercise daily to keep muscles strong. Weakened muscles do not adequately protect the joints. When joints are painful, swimming and water aerobics are ideal.

4. Use affected joints only within the limits of their blood supply. Resting during acute episodes, then quickly returning to activity, is very important in preventing chronic disability.

5. Use medications with caution. Analgesics, muscle relaxants, and nonsteroidal anti-inflammatory drugs may help, especially in the acute phase. Steroid therapy can produce dramatic improvement; but in the long run it usually does more harm than good.

6. If joint destruction is advanced, the joint may need to be fused or replaced with an artificial joint. Surgical procedures are available to correct deformities and to repair injuries.

NOTES

Creeping Fat

Americans are among the fattest people on earth.

Americans are among the fattest people on earth. Obesity is one of our leading public health problems. So serious is this disease that 36 million people are at significant medical risk.

That's frightening. No wonder weight-loss diets are so popular!

Yes, and far too many people fall prey to fads and eating plans that offer quick results. Like a conditioned reflex, extra pounds spell d-i-e-t to most people. A recent survey found that 40 to 50 percent of Americans between the ages of 35 and 59 were on some kind of diet at any given time.

The sad truth is that unless people make lasting changes in their lifestyles and choose healthful foods on a regular basis, their efforts are largely wasted. Up to 90 percent of dieters regain their lost weight within a year, and often with a bonus. Constantly losing and regaining weight is frustrating and demoralizing, and does more damage than good.

GIRTH OF A NATION

United States	172
Europe	156
South & Central America	146
Africa	139
Asia	127

The average weight of men and women, in pounds, based on an assumed height of 5'4".

Would it be better just to stay fat?

For many people, remaining overweight would be less harmful than endlessly playing the rhythm game of girth control. Before running up the white flag of surrender, however, take a careful look

> "When you sit down to eat with a ruler, observe what is set before you.... Don't be greedy for the delicacies he serves; food that looks good may actually be harmful."
> —Proverbs 23:1-3 Clear Word.

at the health risks of being overweight.*

When compared with people of normal weight, obese people are:

- three times more likely to suffer from heart disease.
- four times more likely to suffer from high blood pressure.
- five times more likely to develop diabetes and elevated blood cholesterols.
- at higher risk of developing cancer of the colon, rectum, prostate, breast, cervix, uterus, and ovaries, and of suffering osteoarthritis and low back pain.

Overweight people are like ticking bombs waiting for one or more of these diseases to explode in their lives. In addition, extra weight affects self-image. In today's appearance-oriented society, being overweight can be a great psychological burden.

What causes obesity?

The key to the problem is calories—too many of them. Overweight happens when you eat more calories than your body can use. Whether calories come from fat, protein, sugar, or starch, the leftovers are turned into fat. Some of this fat floats around in the blood, plastering and gradually plugging vital oxygen-carrying arteries.

The rest of the leftover fat ends up in the body's central fat bank, located around the midsection. As the central fat bank overflows, embarrassing branch offices often pop up in other parts of the body. For every 3,500 excess calories received by the body, one pound of fat is placed on deposit.

Would losing just a few pounds do any good?

The answer is yes. Excess fat relates so directly to health that a little bit goes a long way. A 10 percent weight reduction in men 35 to 55 years of age will result in a 20 percent decrease in coronary heart disease. On the other hand, a 10 percent increase in weight produces a 30 percent increase in coronary disease. This is just one example of many such relationships. Every pound counts, one way or the other.

Excess weight lays the foundation for nearly every degenerative disease except osteoporosis.

*Obesity, by definition, is being 20 percent or more above ideal weight. Being 10 to 19 percent above ideal weight is usually termed overweight.

0 Basic Habits to Form for Permanent Weight Control

1. **Eat lots of foods "as grown."** These are the unrefined complex carbohydrate foods, high in fiber and nutrients, yet low in calories and price, and devoid of cholesterol.
2. **Never skip breakfast.** A hot multigrain cereal with fruit is great!
3. **Eat three meals a day** at regular times.
4. **Eat slowly.** Take time to enjoy your food.
5. **End your main meal with a piece of fruit.** Save desserts for special treats.
6. **Skip snacks and night munchies** (or eat a piece of fruit).
7. **Drink plenty of water** instead of juice or sodas.
8. **Exercise daily** (30-60 minutes, or 10,000 steps a day).
9. **Allow no harmful substances into your body** (alcohol, tobacco, caffeine, drugs, etc.).
10. **Develop hobbies**—music, books, sports, etc.

Extra Weight Shortens Life!

Every extra pound shaves off about one month from your life span. Sixty extra pounds, therefore, could cost you five years!

Think Long-term

Improving your health and energy is a more successful motivator over time than wanting to get thin for a wedding or a college reunion. Personalize the risk of being overweight. Pay attention to your blood pressure, your blood cholesterol and triglycerides, and your family history of disease. Losing just 10 percent of your body weight can significantly improve your health.

Fat, regardless of location, causes the same health problems.

What are some positive ways to deal with obesity?

The strategy for successful weight control is threefold:

- Eat more food "as grown," simply prepared, without all the sugar, oil, and salt.
- Increase the rate at which calories are burned by increasing physical activity and muscle size.
- Make the above two lifestyle practices a permanent part of life.

Begin by eating generous amounts of high-fiber foods, such as whole grains, vegetables, fruits, potatoes, yams, and beans. Omit as much fat and sugar from the diet as possible. Cut back on refined and processed foods and snacks. These engineered taste sensations are stuffed with calories and depleted of nutrients. Kick the "crinkly bag" habit!

Use animal products, such as meat, eggs, ice cream, and cheese, very sparingly. They have no fiber and are loaded with fat. You really don't need them at all!

This kind of eating plan, plus a brisk daily walk, will help you lose one to two pounds a week.

You can fight creeping fat and push up your energy level. You can improve your digestion and feel good every day. Begin right now!

NOTES

Application

Being overweight hurts your self-image and lays the foundation for many diseases. The secret of lasting weight loss begins with eating generous amounts of high-fiber foods while limiting animal products and refined foods. Combine this with a brisk, daily walk, and you will easily drop those extra pounds at a healthy rate of one to two pounds a week.

Different Problem, Same Cure

Over and over you've heard the same advice: Change your lifestyle to prevent heart disease, stroke, hypertension, diabetes, and a host of other life-shortening diseases.

Why do all these problems have the same solution? Because a diet of whole foods, very low in fat, sugar, salt, and cholesterol, is not a gimmick or fad—it's the diet your body was designed for.

It should come as no surprise, then, that the same diet that keeps your arteries clean and reduces the risk of cancer also helps you lose weight—and keep it off for good.

Fats Make Fat

Ounce for ounce the American diet packs a lot of calories. That's because it's high in fat. Look at the comparison: a gram of fat contains more than twice the calories of an equal amount of protein or carbohydrate.

CALORIES PER GRAM

Fat	9
Alcohol	7
Carbohydrate	4
Protein	4

Esau's Pottage *(Genesis 25:34)*

1/3 c brown rice (raw)
4 c water
1 c sautéed onions
1 c lentils
herbs to taste: marjoram, thyme, *Mrs. Dash*

Add ingredients to Crockpot and cook until tender. Add herbs shortly before serving. Garnish with parsley and slices of red bell pepper.

Count Those Calories

Which of the following contains the most calories: Salties, Vegi-o's, or Yummies? Compute, figure out the total calories per food, and fill in the blanks:

FDA'S PACKAGING GUIDELINES

	Saltines	Vegi-o's	Yummies
Carbohydrate	8 gm	4 gm	2 gm
Protein	4 gm	5 gm	5 gm
Fat	2 gm	5 gm	7 gm
Weight	14 gm	14 gm	14 gm
Total Calories			

Eat More, Weigh Less

If you picked Yummies, you were correct. Although the weight was the same for all three, Yummies carry a higher proportion of that weight as fat. As a result, a serving of Yummies contains 91 calories while Vegi-o's carry 81 and Saltines only 66 calories.

Keep this in mind when you choose your food. You don't have to eat less to cut calories. In fact, if you choose foods that are high in unrefined complex carbohydrates and low in fat, you can actually eat *more* than ever and still lose weight. That's good news for anyone who thinks going hungry is the only way to get thin. To get thin, you have to eat more, but of the right foods!

Your Challenge

When you shop, check the labels to see how much fat, carbohydrate, and protein the foods you buy contain. Choose those that are high in unrefined complex carbohydrates and low in calorie-dense fats. Remember, if you eat products that carry most of their weight as fat, soon you will be doing the same.

The Cooler Delusion

They look like soft drinks, taste like soft drinks, and are sold like soft drinks. But there the similarity stops. These drinks contain more alcohol than a beer or a glass of wine, and they carry more calories.

Are you talking about flavored coolers? They look so attractive, so healthy!

That's the strategy. These coolers come in a rainbow of colors that people associate with fruit juices. In fact, the containers and carrying packs are often plastered with pictures of fresh fruit even though some contain no fruit or fruit juice at all.

What's more, coolers taste sweet and fizzy, like soft drinks. The alcohol taste is disguised, making them attractive to people who do not ordinarily drink alcohol. Then, too, coolers are packaged, not like other types of alcoholic beverages, but like soft drinks.

Do coolers carry less risk than other alcoholic beverages?

The worst part of the cooler caper is the illusion that coolers are low in alcohol. They're not. Coolers average 6 percent alcohol by volume, whereas beers average 4 percent.

And because coolers usually come in 12-ounce bottles, the amount of alcohol in a serving can exceed that of a gin and tonic (with one ounce of liquor) or a glass of wine served at dinner.

How are coolers affecting today's young people?

Teens, especially teenage girls, are attracted to coolers. They like the name; it suggests a light, refreshing drink. And they like the taste. "Coolers are a hazard for kids because they're so easy to drink," says Diane Purcell of Chicago's Parkside Medical Services. "You can go

ALCOHOL is closely linked with virtually every negative aspect of society: suicide, violent crime, birth defects, industrial accidents, domestic and sexual abuse, disease, homelessness, and death. It is the number one drug problem for people from all walks of life. It knows no racial, ethnic, social, or economic barriers.

—*National Council on Alcohol and Drug Dependency*

Alcohol Facts

- Two of every three adults drink.
- Alcohol is a factor in more than 100,000 deaths, including nearly half of America's murders, suicides, and accidental deaths.
- It's estimated that 32 percent of all patients in general hospital beds are being treated for complications of alcohol-related problems.
- The economic costs to society of alcoholism and alcohol abuse are estimated at more than $200 billion a year, including $31 billion for treatment.

from lemonade to a lemon cooler in one easy step. You don't have to acquire a taste for alcohol."

How serious is alcohol use among teens?

A recent survey revealed that at least 40 percent of sixth graders, and up to 80 percent of junior and senior high school students, have tried wine coolers. Of all 12- to 17-year-olds, 37 percent currently use alcohol. And 5 million American teens already have serious problems stemming from alcohol use. For them, alcohol is the most frequently used drug.

Are these kids in danger of becoming adult alcoholics?

Many kids are already alcoholics by the time they reach adulthood. Others are well on their way.

When it comes to alcohol, people carry their habits into adult life. And there are already 12 million adult alcoholics and 8 million more who have drinking-related problems. In general, half of all fatal auto accidents involve alcohol. Alcohol-related car crashes are the number one killer of

Two of every three high school seniors have drunk alcohol within the past month, and 5 percent drink daily; 40 percent of sixth graders have tasted wine coolers.

teens. Unless we can help our teenagers, things aren't going to get better.

Alcohol exacts a heavy price from personal health. Alcohol promotes high blood pressure and is directly toxic to heart muscle. Alcohol increases the risk of stroke, sudden death from heart arrhythmias and diseased heart muscle, congestive heart failure, cirrhosis and cancer. Alcohol also increases morbidity and hospitalization and reduces the drinker's years of useful life. And it ravages the lives of family and friends.

Perhaps the saddest statistics to emerge in recent years are those of damaged babies permanently mentally deficient as a result of their parents' alcohol use.

How can we best protect our young people?

The challenge to stay drug-and-alcohol-free is greater now than ever for America's teenagers. It is during their early teen years that most will face the critical decision of how they will personally respond to these issues. Each day billboards, magazines, and television, as well as many movies, tell our kids that drinking alcohol is synonymous with being accepted and having a good time. And peer pressure is enormous.

Yet today's youth can be very discerning. Most hold strong

> ## The Wise Man summed it up long ago:
>
> "Wine is a mocker and beer a brawler: whoever is led astray by them is not wise." (Proverbs 20:1)

ideals about what is right and fair, yet they need guidance in making right choices.

- Their immediate need is for education—an honest, reliable, credible source of information. To be effective, this education must start early, during the elementary years.
- Youth need support and encouragement—from grandparents, teachers, churches, mentors, and positive role models. This support must include the availability of positive activities to fill their free time, such as part-time jobs, sports, hobbies, crafts, library use, clubs such as Boy and Girl Scouts, and opportunities to work as community service volunteers.
- But most important of all is a good parental example. Nothing is more powerful than this! And the statistics show it. Young people who grow up in nonalcoholic homes are much less inclined to have problems with alcohol when they reach adulthood.

> "Don't let wine tempt you, even though it looks rich and red and sparkles in your glass. In the end it will bite like a snake and shoot its poison into your veins —Proverbs 23:31-33 *Clear Word*

How Alcohol Affects Your Body

YOUR BRAIN—Alcohol, even in small amounts, causes irreparable damage to brain cells; some die, and others are altered.

YOUR HEART—Alcohol increases the risk of hypertension, stroke, and damage to the heart muscle.

YOUR LUNGS—Alcohol depresses respiratory functions.

YOUR REPRODUCTIVE SYSTEM—In men, alcohol can damage cells in the testes, causing impotence, sterility, and possibly enlarged breasts. In women, alcohol can cause irregular menstrual cycles and malfunctioning of the ovaries. Alcohol has also been linked to birth defects in infants and to fetal alcohol syndrome.

YOUR LIVER—Because your liver must filter alcohol from the blood, alcohol affects the liver more than any other organ of your body:

- Excess calories in alcohol are stored as fat in the liver.
- Functioning liver cells die from alcoholic poisoning.
- Scar tissue replaces dead cells, causing cirrhosis.

YOUR IMMUNE SYSTEM—Alcohol weakens the body's defense against infection and breast cancer.

Alcohol extracts a heavy price on personal health. This goes for teens as well as adults. Young people who grow up in non-alcoholic homes are less likely to have problems with alcohol when they reach adulthood. The example of a parent can make a big difference.

The World's Most Abused Drug

Alcohol is not just a problem for young people; it's the greatest drug problem in the world for all ages. In the United States it's second only to tobacco on the list, "Most Deadly Drugs."

Despite the dangers, everyone in our society comes into contact with alcoholic beverages. If nothing else, we are exposed to commercials on television singing the praises of one brew after another.

Alcohol and Nutrition

Throughout this book we have urged you to avoid highly refined products that are high in calories but low in nutrition. Alcohol certainly falls into this category. With every gram of alcohol containing 7 calories, it comes in calorie-density right after fat, which carries 9 calories per gram. And those calories add up fast: Two cans of beer, for example, carry 300 calories; two jiggers of 100 proof whiskey, 250 calories; two glasses of dessert wine pack 280 calories—and they are all empty calories, providing none of the nutrients your body requires.

For men, alcohol accounts for 9 percent of the calories in the American diet. No wonder we are overfed and undernourished.

Your Challenge

Make this "ban the booze" week at your house. You should be able to get through it without any sort of urge or discomfort.

If you can't, you need to seriously consider who is the master: you or the alcohol. If you can get through the week with no problems, why not quit altogether? It will help keep your weight under control, improve your nutrition, and set a good example for the young people in your life.

Alcohol and Young People

Young people ages 14 to 24 account for more than 8,000 alcohol-related fatalities—about a third of the annual total.

Those Lost Years

"When you're a teenager, it's hard to think of time ever being short; it's hard to realize what a precious commodity time is."

NOTES

_____

_____

_____

_____

"Don't drink wine because it's too easy to get drunk."
—Ephesians 5:18 Clear Word

The Deadliest Drug

"Smoking is the single most preventable cause of death in America."
—U.S. Surgeon General

Smoking is not only hazardous to your health—it can be hazardous to your job prospects as well. Twice as many smokers are out of work as nonsmokers. Though few will admit it, most employers would reject a smoker competing for a job with an equally qualified nonsmoker.

Don't you think the risks of smoking are being exaggerated?

No way! For example, smokers at Dow Chemical, when compared to nonsmokers, had six days more absenteeism, eight days more disability, and 12 percent more illness, costing the company $8,945 more per smoker per year.

The hard facts consistently point to tobacco as the deadliest drug in the world. On average it kills about 450,000 Americans a year—more than all who die from AIDS, street drugs, fires, car crashes, and homicides combined. This includes 46,500 involuntary smokers—persons forced to breathe secondhand smoke.

How does smoking cause lung cancer?

Normally your lungs' air passages are lined with millions of tiny hairs called cilia. These cilia act like little brooms protecting the air tubes by sweeping dusts, tar, and other foreign materials gradually upward, like escalators, until they can be spit out.

Every time a blast of tobacco smoke hits these cilia, however, they slow down, and soon stop moving. As a result, the trapped tars from the tobacco smoke begin boring into the cells lining the air tubes. Over time, this constant irritation turns some of the cells cancerous.

This transformation takes many years. But once it begins, the cancer steadily eats its way deeper into the lung. By the time it is discovered, it's usually too late. Is lung cancer the leading cause of death in smokers?

> "Do you not know that your body is a temple? Therefore honor God with your body." —1 Corinthians 6:19, 20

No. Tobacco causes 125,500 lung cancer deaths per year in the United States. In contrast, smoking is responsible for 135,000 heart attacks and strokes. Plus 45,000 who took in the smoke second hand as involuntary smokers.

The nicotine and carbon monoxide in tobacco smoke are the main culprits that promote vascular disease. Nicotine constricts small arteries depriving the heart, brain, lungs, and other important areas of vital oxygen. Nicotine also produces a sense of relaxation and well-being—smoking's main appeal. But nicotine is also addictive.

Carbon monoxide interferes directly with the ability of red blood cells to carry oxygen. This causes shortness of breath, lack of endurance, and acceleration of atherosclerosis (narrowing and hardening of the arteries).

That's a lot of bad news. Is there more?

Unfortunately there is a lot more.

- Smokers have much more cancer of the mouth, larynx, esophagus, pancreas, bladder, kidneys, and cervix than do nonsmokers.
- Emphysema gradually destroys

"Every cigarette smoked takes 13 minutes off a person's life span."

lung tissue, producing death by suffocation. In the United States 86,000 of these grisly deaths occur each year as a result of smoking.
- Ulcers of the stomach and duodenum are 60 percent more common in smokers.

- Smoking pulls calcium out of the skeleton, accelerating the bone-thinning process known as osteoporosis.
- Smoking during pregnancy has an adverse effect on fetal development and increases the risk of death after birth by up to 35 percent.

If a person has smoked heavily for a long time, does it pay to quit?

About 85 percent of lung cancers and 50 percent of bladder cancers could be prevented if people simply stopped smoking.

Smokers who quit begin to heal almost immediately. As the nicotine and carbon monoxide leave the body, the smoking-related risk for heart disease decreases dramatically. Although the risk for cancer decreases more slowly, the danger lessens as the weeks and months go by.

Merchants of Death

During the past five years American tobacco companies have tripled their export of cigarettes. As a result, Asia and Africa have become the newest killing fields.

Legalized Death

Cigarettes are among the world's most profitable drugs. They are also the only legal ones that, if used as intended, turn most of their users into addicts and kill every second smoker.

There are other payoffs to quitting: a sense of victory, increased self-esteem, pleasant breath, better-tasting food, increased endurance, improved health and energy, a feeling of well-being, and freedom from an inconvenient, unpopular, and costly habit. Quitting may also open the way to more job opportunities.

Americans often overreact to the most trivial of risks while ignoring much more substantial threats to their health and safety. For example, every second smoker will die from some disease directly connected to the habit. Smokers will also lose an average of 14 years from their normal life expectancy, or 13 minutes for every cigarette smoked. Yet many people react more forcefully to evidence of a one-in-a-million risk of getting cancer from chemicals found in drinking water!

It's time to get life back into perspective. The biggest favor you can do your body is to kick the habit and freely breathe clean air again.

Did You Know …

That smoking kills 1,200 Americans a day and costs $2.1 billion a week in extra health-care and insurance costs, while the state and federal government collect $30 billion a year in tobacco taxes.

How Smoking Kills

Tobacco use kills and maims primarily by promoting vascular diseases and various cancers.

Vascular diseases
- Heart attacks—smoking is responsible for 30 percent of the annual 550,000 U.S. coronary deaths.
- Stroke—responsible for 25 percent of the annual strokes.
- Peripheral vascular disease—some 90 percent of leg and thigh blockages occur in smokers.

Cancers
- Lung—85 percent because of smoking.
- Bladder and kidneys—three times more frequent in smokers.
- Mouth, larynx, esophogus—two to 25 times more prevalent in smokers.

Tobacco is the deadliest drug in the world. In the United States alone it kills about 450,000 people a year. The biggest favor people can do for themselves is to break the smoking habit.

You Can Do It!

Kicking the Habit

The first step in breaking any habit is to decide that you are going to change. It's not enough just to want to change or to imagine that you will change someday. Breaking an addiction to tobacco requires positive commitment.

You have everything to gain by kicking the habit—longer life, better health, more vitality, fewer medical expenses … and the air is fresher, food tastes better, wallets are fatter, age is longer, life is sweeter!

Reasons to Quit Smoking

Here are a few reasons that have convinced thousands to quit last year:

1. Quitting is the single most important thing you can do for your health and longevity.
2. Reduced risk of heart disease, stroke, and cancer of the lungs, mouth, throat, pancreas, bladder, kidneys, and cervix.
3. Reduced risk of emphysema and osteoporosis.
4. Elimination of the risk posed to the smoker's family from secondhand smoke.
5. Less chance of a smoker's children and grandchildren smoking.
6. Better breath, whiter teeth, and fewer wrinkles.
7. Less time spent sick: more physical endurance.
8. Lower medical and insurance costs.

The list goes on, and it grows every year as we learn more about the harmful effects of tobacco.

NOTES

Are You Wired?

Nine out of 10 North Americans take a psychotropic (mind-altering) drug daily. The culprit? Everyday, ordinary, over-the-counter caffeine.

How can that be? Explain.

Do you know many people who don't drink at least one cup of coffee a day? Or tea? Or take an extra-strength pain reliever? Or guzzle down a cola? Although caffeine-free sodas are available, they are favored mainly for children and for people with medical problems that are affected by caffeine.

But I need a lift now and then! And caffeine isn't addictive, is it?

An addictive substance produces observable and measurable physical and mental effects when it is withdrawn. In this sense, even small doses of caffeine, taken regularly over time, will usually produce some degree of addiction.

A good way to check yourself is to stop all caffeine intake for a few days. The most common physical withdrawal symptom is headache, varying from mild to severe. Sometimes a migraine is triggered. Other physical manifestations include feelings of exhaustion, lack of appetite, nausea, and vomiting. These symptoms may last from one to five days.

Psychological withdrawal can be even harder. Depression may occur. People become accustomed to reaching for the pick-me-up throughout the day. The urge can be compared to the desire for a cigarette—it may be difficult to resist.

Everyone wants to hear that coffee is good for us. But let's get real. We love the rich aroma and taste of coffee, and we do like something hot in the morning. But we're not fooling anyone—what we want is the buzz, the caffeine.

Does caffeine damage the body?

- Most obvious is an overstimulated nervous system with tremors, nervousness, anxiety, and sleep problems. In time these symptoms give way to chronic fatigue, lack of energy, and persistent insomnia.
- Caffeinated beverages can cause stomach irritation. While additives are primarily responsible for this effect, caffeine itself has a constricting effect on blood vessels. It can thus interfere with digestion.
- Caffeinated drinks stimulate the stomach to excrete excessive acid. This may aggravate ulcers.
- Caffeine has been found to interfere with calcium and iron absorption associated with osteoporosis and anemia.
- Caffeine increases energy by raising blood sugar levels. These, in turn, draw out an insulin response that not only cancels the surge but produces a letdown. This letdown triggers the yo-yo syndrome—reaching for another caffeinated drink, and then another, and yet another.
- Caffeine also irritates the kidneys and acts as a diuretic (increased urine output).

Are there some healthful alternatives to the caffeine high?

When you get up in the morning, follow your hot shower with a blast of cold water and towel off briskly. At work, stand up, stretch, and take a few deep breaths every hour or so. Take a brisk walk at breaktime or during lunch hour. Drink a cup of cold (or hot) water several times a day. Rub a coworker's back and ask for a return favor. Walk to a window and relax your eyes on the distant landscape. Tidy up your work area. All these good things will make you feel better. Look for other creative ways to get a lift without the letdown.

In a crisis, would just a little caffeine really matter?

Occasional small doses of caffeine will hardly make a difference. The trouble is, most of us have a hard time knowing when to stop.

Java Water has grown steadily since it was introduced in 1996. A 17-ounce bottle of this flavorless spring water contains a hefty 140 mg of caffeine. Caffeinated orange juice and lemonade are also popular.

A person can get hooked with a relatively small amount of caffeine if it's on a fairly regular basis.

Caffeine can produce:

- Elevated blood sugar
- Increased blood pressure
- Elevated blood fats (triglycerides)
- Heightened symptoms of PMS
- Tremors, irritability, and nervousness
- Aggravation of anxiety disorders and panic attacks
- Increased stomach acid secretions
- Urinary calcium and magnesium losses
- Insomnia
- Irregular heartbeat
- Increased stimulation of the central nervous system (it overrules the need for rest)

Where Is the Caffeine?

Coffee/Tea
(average)

Cup drip coffee	145 mg
Cup brewed coffee	115 mg
Cup instant coffee	85 mg
Cup decaffeinated	3 mg
1.5-oz. shot espresso	100 mg
Cup hot tea	65 mg
Iced tea (12 oz.)	70 mg

Wake up and smell the caffeine, folks—America's drug of choice is not limited to your morning cup of coffee.

Popular Headache Medications
(1 pill)

Vivarin	100-200 mg
NoDoz	100-200 mg
Excedrin	65 mg
Anacin	40 mg
Plain aspirin	0 mg
Tylenol	0 mg
Cold medications	0-30 mg

Soda
(12-oz. serving)

Monster Drink	120 mg
Java Water	100 mg
Jolt	100 mg
Sugar-free Mr. Pibb	60 mg
Mountain Dew	54 mg
Coke and Diet Coke	45 mg
Pepsi-Cola	40 mg

Chocolate

1 oz. milk chocolate	6 mg
1 oz. unsweetened baking chocolate	25 mg
1/4 cup choc. chips	15 mg
8 oz. chocolate milk	10 mg

Caffeine can be an addictive drug. Regular use over time often produces physical and mental effects when withdrawn. While an occasional small dose of caffeine may not make a difference, heavier use has been linked to health problems.

Are you living drug-free?

Coffee: Food or Drug?

Imagine going to buy coffee at the grocery store and finding the coffee section missing.

"What's going on?" you ask the clerk. "Where is the coffee?"

"Oh, haven't you heard? Coffee has been classified as a drug. The pharmacist sells it now."

Shaking your head in disbelief, you walk across the store to where the pharmacist dispenses medications, drugs, and—caffeinated beverages.

The pharmacist smiles at you knowingly. "You look like you're here for some coffee. I can tell from your expression."

You nod and tell him what brand you would like.

"That's fine," he says. "No prescription necessary—I just need to type up the warning label."

"Warning label?"

"That's right. Take a look at it."

> **Warning:** This drink contains caffeine. Possible side effects include addiction, tremors, nervousness, anxiety, insomnia, chronic fatigue, lack of energy, stomach irritation, vomiting, interference with calcium and iron absorption, and the aggravation of ulcers.

He hands you the coffee, but you decline. "No thanks," you say. "I think I've changed my mind."

Are You an Addict?

You could be a caffeine addict without even knowing it.

One way to find out if you are addicted is to stop all caffeine intake for a week. If you're hooked, chances are good that you will notice such physical symptoms as headache, lack of appetite, and nausea, which can last from one to five days. Psychologically, you may feel down and listless, and of course, there will be a strong urge for your favorite beverage.

Breaking the Habit

If you find you're a caffeine fiend, here are a few things you can do to ease through withdrawal.

1. Gradually reduce the amount of caffeine.
2. Replace it with decaffeinated coffee and by drinking more water.
3. Slow down your daily activities.
4. Exercise in the fresh air.
5. Get the support of others around you.
6. Reward yourself for taking such a positive step.

Your Challenge

Cut down on caffeinated drinks—tea, coffee, and colas—and eventually skip them altogether. See how you fare. At the end of a week, review this material and give serious consideration to making your body a caffeine-free zone.

NOTES

Spiders and Sledgehammers

"I would lose one third to one half of my patients if I didn't prescribe valium or similar drugs."
—*a frustrated physician*

The way some people use drugs makes no more sense than using a sledgehammer to kill a spider. It's not just prescription drugs that pose problems, either. Common over-the-counter drugs can have unpleasant—even dangerous—side effects.

You must be exaggerating.

I wish I were! Take something as common as aspirin, for instance. Many people down it at the least sign of a headache, flu, or fever. As a matter of fact, every 24 hours Americans consume 45 tons of this drug!

Yet every year 10,000 people will be severely poisoned by aspirin or a related product. What's more, aspirin is known to promote stomach ulcers. It has also been associated with Reye's syndrome, an often fatal disease in children, and in older people it can trigger a hemorrhagic stroke.

Acetaminophen and ibuprofen, other common painkillers, can cause skin rashes and—in extreme cases—kidney and liver damage.

But prescription drugs are safe when you follow directions, right?

In the medical world new and more effective wonder drugs are being discovered and introduced almost daily, while older ones are improved and refined. Yet the perfect drug still eludes us—the one that will do its job with absolutely no deleterious side effects.

Consider blood pressure drugs. They are the most widely used prescription medications on the market and among the more effective ones. Yet they carry a host of side effects. These can include weakness, fatigue, drowsiness, headache, mental depression,

> **"Show me the way I should go, for to you I lift up my soul."**
> —Psalm 143:8

dizziness, bloating, sweating, indigestion, unstable emotional states, slurred speech, raised cholesterol levels, and impotence. People who need these drugs often must test several different kinds before they find one they can tolerate.

The point is, no drug is completely safe. Even life-saving antibiotics carry potential problems, such as nausea, vomiting, diarrhea, allergic reactions, and yeast infections.

Why, then, are people so anxious to take drugs?

While most of today's diseases respond to lifestyle measures (such as a better diet and regular exercise), physicians who advocate these principles often find themselves rowing upstream. Most people are impatient. They want quick fixes rather

Many sedatives and tranquilizers are addictive when used over time.

than real solutions. If one physician doesn't produce the desired prescription, they often find another one who will.

Simply put, people today too often want to believe there is a magic potion for their problem. With an almost childlike faith we swallow drugs to pep us up, to calm us down, to regulate our weight, and to ward off almost every conceivable symptom.

So why risk taking any drug?

When physicians prescribe drugs, they must always balance risk against need. For instance, with a serious bacterial infection, the risk you run by taking an antibiotic is usually outweighed by the risk you run if you don't take it.

If you have a tension headache, on the other hand, you'd probably be better off taking a brisk walk or a nap.

What are some guidelines for using drugs intelligently?

A good rule of thumb is to reserve drugs for specific, identifiable needs

rescription Drugs

You won't have the answers if you don't ask the questions. These are the questions you need to ask:

- What is the full name and strength of the medication?
- How will the medicine help me?
- What are the risks?
- What side effects can I expect?
- How, when, and for how long do I take it?
- What should I do if I miss a dose?
- Is there written information I can take with me?
- Is there a non-drug alternative for my problem?

This is the information you need to provide:

- About all other medicines you are taking, including self-medications with non-prescription drugs, such as aspirin, vitamins, or cold/allergy pills.
- If cost is a concern to you.
- If you have any allergies or medical conditions, and how or if they are being treated.

Safety First

Many people believe medicines sold without prescription are safe and have no side effects. NO DRUG IS COMPLETELY SAFE. For example, acetaminophen (Tylenol) and ibuprofen (Advil, Motrin) used regularly for long periods of time have been shown to double the risk of kidney cancer and triple the risk of kidney damage.

Legalized Death

Cigarettes are among the world's most profitable drugs. They are the delivery system of Nicotine. But they are also the only legal ones that, if used as intended, turn most of their users into addicts and kill every second smoker.

that can't be met by lesser measures. Don't use a big-gun medicine like antibiotics, for instance, for a flyswatter problem like a head cold.

Likewise, a warm bath or a cup of herb tea is better than a sleeping pill if you can't get to sleep. And if you don't want to go to sleep, a cold shower or a brisk walk is better for you than a wake-up pill or cup of coffee.

When you do take a drug, be sure you know exactly what it's supposed to do. Understand its risks and side effects, how and when to take it, and the signs of overdosage. Don't mix medicines, and don't risk psychological dependence or physical addiction by taking any drug longer than needed. If you have more than one doctor, make sure your main doctor knows all the medications you are taking.

In short, give drugs the respect they deserve. Save them for the times they are truly needed.

It's time to stop hitting spiders with sledgehammers.

NOTES

_____

_____

_____

_____

_____

_____

_____

_____

_____

_____

_____

_____

_____

_____

Application

Many people have a childlike faith in drugs and medicines. They take them for every conceivable ailment. But using big-gun medicines for flyswatter problems, or for problems that should be solved by lifestyle measures, can leave you tired, depleted, and depressed. Use drugs sparingly and with care.

Pain Is a Warning

Too many people run to the medicine cabinet whenever they feel the slightest ache or pain. They don't realize that pain often acts as a warning system telling us something is wrong.

We may be eating too much, drinking too much, smoking too much, or taking on obligations beyond our capacities. When pain is blocked by drugs, we ignore these causes rather than changing the behaviors that are causing the pain in the first place. This kind of neglect sets the stage for more serious diseases.

Two Categories of Drugs

Some drugs attack the cause of a problem; others mainly relieve symptoms.

If you take any medications, list them in the spaces below. Write a C next to those that attack the cause of the problem. Put an S by those that simply help relieve symptoms.

_____

_____

_____

_____

_____

_____

_____

_____

_____

_____

Your Challenge

Don't go running to the medicine cabinet for every little ache and pain. The "cure" is often worse than the problem. When you must take a drug, be sure you get the answers to the questions on the drug checklist (see page 81).

Upper Drugs	Downer Drugs
Caffeine	Tranquilizers
Tobacco	Sedatives
Some diet pills	Alcohol
Amphetamines	Tobacco

The Positives

Sense of well-being	Relaxes
Decreased fatigue	Relieves anxiety
Sharpens mind	False sense of peacefulness

The Negatives

Only temporary	Temporary effect
Depletes resources	Solves no problems
Premature aging	Depression
Depression	

Modern medicine is a three-legged stool. Drugs and surgery are two legs—the third is what people can do for themselves:

- Healthful lifestyle changes
- Regular active exercise
- Pursuit of spiritual goals

GOD SAID: "I give you every seed-bearing plant on the face of the whole earth and every tree that has fruit with seed in it. They will be yours for food." —*Genesis 1:29*

Understanding Food

- Digestion
- Starch
- Sugar
- Bread
- Protein
- Milk
- Meat
- Fat
- Cholesterol
- Fiber
- Salt
- Vitamins, Minerals, Herbs
- Phytochemicals and Antioxidants

What Follows the Swallows

Water gives your body an internal shower.

Digestion is the process by which the body breaks down food into its major constituents, which are proteins, fats, and carbohydrates. They carry the food's energy to tthe body. The gut digests each in an orderly fashion, yet at different rates. It digests simple carbohydrates (sugars) quickly, while fats take longer. Proteins and complex carbohydrates (starches) fall somewhere in between, depending on their fiber content.

Is there some benefit in eating a starch food, for instance, at one meal and a protein food at a different time?

Nature doesn't support this idea. All plant foods and some animal foods are combinations of carbohydrate, protein, and fat. Beans and peas, for example, have quite a bit of protein, and corn has a fair percentage of fat.

To get a pure carbohydrate meal, you would need to eat white sugar or the starchy residue that's left after removing the gluten from white flour. A pure protein meal could be egg whites or dry cottage cheese curds. For the fat meal, a few tablespoons of butter or cooking oil would do. Pure foods, in this sense, don't occur in nature, but they can be manufactured.

How does the stomach handle these different food constituents?

During digestion sugars and starches of the carbohydrates become glucose, fats become fatty acids, and proteins become amino acids. The blood then can pick up these smaller substances from the intestines and distribute them.

> "Eat for strength and not just to dine and get drunk."
> —Ecclesiastes 10:17 Clear Word

Only a part of digestion occurs in the stomach. The rest occurs in the mouth and intestines. In an amazingly orderly fashion, carbohydrate digestion begins in the mouth with the saliva and continues in the stomach. Protein digestion begins in the stomach and continues in the intestines. Fat is largely digested in the intestines.

Does the acidity or alkalinity of foods affect this process?

The stomach has three basic functions:

- It breaks food particles down to a more uniform size by muscular action.
- It brings the food mass to the needed consistency by adding or absorbing fluid.
- It brings the stomach contents to the necessary degree of acidity by secreting acidic digestive juices. This phase accomplishes

The flavor of food is appreciated through taste buds, nearly 9,000 of which are located on the human tongue. Each taste bud connects with about 50 nerve fibers.

those parts of digestion that require an acid medium.

When the stomach contents go on to the intestines, they become alkalinized by juices that the pancreas secretes. The digestive process is completed in the intestines.

Don't some foods bog down this process?

Foods high in fats are the worst offenders. The body cannot digest fats until they are alkalinized and emulsified by the intestinal juices (much as the grease on your hands cannot be removed until it is emulsified with soap and hot water).

But the body has protective mechanisms that meter the fat from the stomach to the intestines so that the emulsification process isn't overwhelmed. If the amount of fat in a meal is not large, it will make little difference in digestion time. But a typical Western meal, because of its high fat con-

Do you ever think about what happens to your food after you swallow it?

Most of us take our digestive system very much for granted. We eat whatever we want, whenever we want. But how does our body handle the food it's given?

One of our worst habits relates to the TIME we eat.

It's not just WHAT we eat, but WHEN we eat. The digestive machinery works best when given time to digest one meal before the next meal comes along.

Drinking fluids with meals dilutes the digestive juices— and slows down digestion. It is best to drink water about two hours after a meal, and up to 15 minutes preceding it.

tent, may need four to five hours, or longer, to pass through the stomach.

Is there an ideal balance of foods?

The body can handle three or four kinds of whole plant foods with maximum efficiency and minimum stress. A more complex meal takes longer to digest and exacts a higher energy price from the body.

Eating snacks between meals disrupts the orderly digestive processes and stresses the stomach. Digestive problems will be slight if the stomach is presented with a simple meal, allowed to digest it, and then is given time to rest before adding more food. Ideally, meals should be four to five hours apart.

You mean we shouldn't eat anything between meals?

Take a drink of water. Water requires no digestion. It passes right through, giving everything a good rinse. If you just must have something more, choose a piece of fresh fruit or munch on some raw veggies.

One last thought . . .

Swallowing seems so easy we take it for granted without any further thought. But digestion is actually a very complicated physiological action. It requires the carefully coordinated efforts of 30 muscles, or group of muscles — and once it's begun, you can't stop it at will.

NOTES

_____

_____

_____

_____

_____

_____

_____

_____

_____

Application

How do you spell relief? If you are like most North Americans, you spell it D-O-L-L-A-R-S. Each year we spend millions on pills and potions to quiet our angry stomachs. A better way would be: stop overloading your stomach and give it the rest it needs.

Sweetening a Sour Stomach

How often does your stomach protest?

__ Never

__ Several times a year

__ Several times a month

__ Weekly

__ Every day

If you frequently have indigestion or an upset stomach, and your physician has ruled out more serious problems, it may be your eating habits that are causing you grief.

Answer the following questions with a Yes or No.

1. ___ *Do you have regular eating times?*

    Your body thrives on a regular schedule, not only of eating, but of waking, sleeping, and exercise.

2. ___ *Do you often eat between meals?*

    When new food shows up in a stomach that is already working, digestion must slow down until the system deals with the new arrival.

    Imagine a washing machine working on a load of clothes. If you come by every 10 minutes, turn the dial back, and dump in more clothes, you would never finish a load. A washing machine, just like your stomach, needs time to finish its cycle.

3. ___ *Are your meals spaced four to five hours apart?*

    Spacing meals several hours apart allows the stomach to work at its own pace. Food from one meal is completely digested before the next one arrives.

4. ___ *Do you drink coffee?*

    Coffee, even decaf, contains substances that can irritate the lining of the stomach. Too much of this substance can send your stomach into rebellion.

5. ___ *Do you eat right before going to bed?*

    The stomach, like the rest of your body, needs rest. A meal or snack late in the evening forces it to work overtime.

Dealing With Gas

Many people adjusting to a high-fiber diet experience problems with intestinal gas. This is especially true when beans are on the menu. Here are some suggestions that can help:

- For occasional intestinal gas, try some pharmaceutical-grade charcoal. It adsorbs gas and provides a measure of relief. It is available as powder, tablets, syrup, or capsules and is sold over the counter.
- To reduce gas caused by cooked dried beans, try soaking them overnight, discarding the soak water, and replacing it with fresh water for cooking.

Your Challenge

Give your stomach a break by spacing meals further apart. Not interrupting the digestive cycle with snacks will sweeten the disposition of a cranky stomach.

The Body's Premium Fuel

S tarchy foods are the superstars of the food galaxy. The scientific community tells us that the road to better health is paved with potatoes, whole-wheat pasta, brown rice, beans, and good bread.

What about protein? Everybody needs protein!

Yes, but not so much. For a long time people assumed that because muscles were predominantly protein we needed to eat a lot of it to be strong. (Bodybuilders still believe that!)

But the body is like a car. Once the car is built, only a few additional parts are needed here and there for maintenance. Similarly, a human adult needs relatively little protein for daily maintenance—about 45 to 60 grams per day. That's about two ounces of pure protein.

What the car does need on a regular basis is good clean gasoline. And carbohydrates are the gasoline of the body, the high-octane fuel that keeps it running smoothly.

Isn't fat also a body fuel?

Fat, in general, is stored fuel, carried as baggage. It's the reserve tank. If the body runs out of carbohydrate fuel, it can dig out the spare stuff. But fat doesn't burn as cleanly as carbohydrates and it's not as energy-efficient.

What are carbohydrates?

Carbohydrates are the sugars and starches in the foods we eat. A lot of people don't understand the relationship between sugars and starches, and the confusion is compounded when terms like *simple carbohydrates and complex carbohydrates* are used.

In general, simple carbohydrates are the sugars and complex carbohydrates are the starches (see chart on page 92). All carbohydrates, both sugars and starches, are broken down by the digestive tract and end up as glucose. The blood absorbs this glucose from the intestines and uses it for energy (fuel). Complex carbohydrates are almost exclusively found in plant foods—in grains, potatoes, beans, and vegetables, and in the many foods made from them, such as bread and pastas.

The sugars—simple carbohydrates—are digested quickly and, unless fiber is present, enter the bloodstream as glucose within minutes. This produces a quick rise in blood sugar, accompanied by an energy increase. But sugar-flooding often causes the pancreas to overreact, sending out a surge of insulin that not only brings the blood sugar back in line but sometimes drops it too low. The result may be an energy dip, often with a feeling of faintness or shakiness. The usual reaction is to grab a snack or a soda to straighten out the problem.

It works, doesn't it?

A better solution would be to eat an apple, pear, or mango. In their natural forms nearly all carbohydrate foods contain liberal amounts of different kinds of fiber. Some kinds are not digested by the body. Instead, they absorb

Wouldn't it be great if you got hooked on foods that made you look and feel great . . . and the more you ate them the healthier you became?

water and form a soft mass in the intestines that acts to slow down the rate of sugar absorption.

Another solution would be to eat more unrefined complex carbohydrates, or starches. Starches are very complex molecules. Much larger than sugar molecules, they take considerably longer to digest. Thus they don't push up the blood sugar level as quickly. Moreover, the fiber content of most unrefined foods is an additional help in leveling out the rates of digestion and the absorption of nutrients.

But aren't starches more fattening than other foods?

Fat is the most fattening food. One gram of fat carries nine calories, while a gram of carbohydrate carries only four calories. Much of the fat we eat goes right into the fat stores of the body.

It's the refining and processing of carbohydrates that causes problems: the volume of the food goes down, while its caloric concentration goes up. It's this caloric density that makes it so easy to eat too many calories! But when carbohydrates are eaten along with their fiber, then you can eat more food yet take in fewer calories.

So what can I eat?

Potatoes, whole-wheat pasta, beans, barley, and brown rice fill people's stomachs without overloading the system with calories. Add a variety of fruits and vegetables, and it's virtually impossible to eat enough to gain weight.

CARBOHYDRATE FAMILY TREE

But top off these healthy foods with butter, gravies, sauces, salad dressings, sour cream, or cheese, and a nutritious, low-calorie food becomes a caloric disaster.

Eating complex carbohydrates "as grown" with their full complement of fiber but without those fatty toppings will not only allow you to eat a greater quantity of food and still lose weight, but provide you with more consistent energy levels and increased endurance. This kind of eating plan will keep your arteries clean and cut your food bill in half. Where can you find a better bargain than that?

The Magic of Food

Wouldn't it be great if you got hooked on foods that made you look and feel great . . . and the more you ate them the healthier you became?

NOTES

Contrary to what many believe, we need less protein and more starch in our diets. Complex carbohydrates found in fruits, vegetables, and grains provide clean-burning energy and increased endurance. Building your diet around these foods helps keep your arteries clean, your food bill low, and your body healthy.

King Potato

The king of the starchy vegetables is the potato. It is filling, nutritious, and tasty. If you have a microwave, it takes only minutes to build a complete meal around this terrific tuber.

Are Potatoes Fattening?

A five-ounce spud contains only 80 calories. The potato's reputation as a fattening food comes from the way it is served—French-fried, baked, and slathered with butter or sour cream. It is the added fat, not the potato itself, that is fattening.

Topping Ideas

Lentils or Beans: Cook up a pot of lentils or beans with some onion and garlic. Ladle them onto a piping-hot baked potato. Served with a green salad and whole-wheat bread, this meal will satisfy even the heartiest appetite.

Salsa: Olé! It might sound a bit unusual, but salsa makes an excellent topping for a baked potato. It's available at many restaurants. Next time you eat out and the server asks, "Butter or sour cream?" say, "Neither." Ask for salsa instead.

Mrs. Dash Seasoning (salt-free blend): Slice a cooked potato into wedges, sprinkle with *Mrs. Dash* (the one with the green cap!) seasonings, and bake until browned. It's the health-conscious chef's answer to French fries.

Leftover Soups and Stews: There are many wonderful recipes for meatless soups and stews that can do double duty as a topping. Get creative and see what you can come up with.

Your Challenge

Add more unrefined complex carbohydrates to your diet. Enjoy whole-grain foods and potatoes. Complex carbohydrates, as they come in nature—unrefined, and usually with a lot of fiber, will fill you up without weighing you down. And they won't cost you an arm and a leg!

NOTES

From Sugar Highs to Sugar Blues

Strip seven pounds of sugar beets of their bulk, fiber, and nutrients, and you will get one pound of "pure" white sugar.

Americans consume an average of 150 pounds of sugars and sweeteners per year for each man, woman, and child. That's almost three fourths of a cup, or some 40 teaspoons of sugar, per person per day.

I don't buy that much sugar. Where does it all come from?

Most of the sugar we consume is hidden sugar. Here are some of the ways sugar slips into our diets:

- *Soft drinks.* Americans average 54 gallons of soft drinks per person per year. This works out to about two sodas per day. One 12-ounce soda may contain 12 teaspoons of sugar.
- *Desserts.* A piece of chocolate cake, for instance, contains 15 teaspoons of sugar; a cup of frozen yogurt has 12 teaspoons.
- *Ready-to-eat cereals.* Some, such as *Shredded Wheat* and *Cheerios,* are excellent. But look at cereals like *Fruit Loops* and *Sugar Smacks,* in which almost half of their calories come from sugar. *This isn't cereal; it's candy!*

And sugar is everywhere. You'll find hidden sugar in foods, such as canned soups, potpies, TV dinners, and ketchup.

Should I check labels for sugar?

Yes, but realize that sugar may also be hidden by giving it a different name. Sucrose, dextrose, lactose, fructose, and maltose, for

FOOD PROCESSING
Concentrates Calories

75 Calories

500 Calories

instance, are all sugars. So are corn syrup, honey, and molasses. Actually, there are more than 100 substances with different names, but they are all sugars.

Doesn't sugar produce quick energy?

Yes, refined, concentrated sugars enter the bloodstream quickly. Up goes the blood sugar, resulting in a quick energy boost—a sugar high.

But the high is only temporary, because it triggers a surge of insulin. This insulin, in turn, brings down the blood sugar into the normal range. But in the absence of the modulating effects of fiber, it sometimes pulls it down too fast and too far.

This falling blood sugar often mimics symptoms of hypoglycemia, producing feelings of weakness, hunger, fatigue, and letdown—the sugar blues. The usual reaction is to reach for another sugary snack, and then another, leading to a sort of grazing all day long.

Here is a better way to handle this: reach out to an apple, a banana, or a bowl of brown rice. The fiber in these foods slows down the absorption of sugar into the bloodstream.

The sugar levels won't jump around so much, your energy will stabilize, and you'll feel satisfied longer.

We can't get enough of the white stuff, even as science warns of obesity and other health risks. Are we off to the sweet hereafter?

Is it true that the body can make sugar out of nearly everything we eat?

Out of everything but fat! For a long time people thought it didn't really matter what they ate, because the body could turn it into whatever it needed. We now know that the way the body processes food, from the time it's eaten until it reaches the bloodstream, makes a great deal of difference.

The body's preferred fuel is glucose, which it makes largely from sugars and starches (carbohydrates). Although fresh fruits can be high in natural sugars, they won't strain the body's blood sugar mechanism if

they are eaten in their natural state with their natural fiber intact. The lesson to be learned: eat more fruit and drink less fruit juice.

Starchy foods have another built-in protective mechanism. Starches are broken down more slowly than sugars into the glucose the body needs. Eating starchy foods, especially unrefined starchy foods with their fiber content intact, along with sugar foods helps stabilize blood sugar levels for extended periods. The ups and downs of the blood sugar curve level off, and the insulin response is activated to a much lesser degree, if at all.

What are some guidelines for eating sweet foods?

Education and moderation are the secrets.

If you have a sweet tooth, see your dentist . . . well, not really, but a sweet tooth can be reeducated. For instance, fruit is sweet, pleasant to the taste, and full of fruit sugars. Practice satisfying your sweet cravings by reaching for a bunch of chilled grapes instead of a doughnut. Sprinkle slices of strawberries and

Are you dragging yourself around?
Snapping at the kids? Feeling shaky and anxious?
It could be low blood sugar—the sugar blues.

Blood sugar dips correspond to energy dips. The person with sugar-rich, poor eating habits alternates between a sense of well-being and an inevitable letdown.

SUGAR

SUGAR CONTENT

Food Portion	Size	Teaspoons of Sugar
Soft drinks	12 oz	8-12
Jello, puddings	1 cup	9
Jelly, Jam	2 Tbsp	5
Pies: apple, berry, cherry	1 slice	10
Chocolate mints	4	6
Marshmallow	10	15
Hard candy	4 oz	20
Grape juice (commercial)	1 cup	7
Fruit cocktail (commercial)	1 cup	8
Doughnut (glazed)	1	6
Angel, pound cake	1 slice)	9
German chocolate cake	1 slice)	15
Ice cream, sherbet	1 cup	6-8
Ice-cream cone only	1 triple	10

Soft drinks are the single biggest source of refined sugar in the U.S. diet.

Scientists are taking a new look at our addiction to sweets, and wonder how giant sodas and oversized candy bars relate specifically to our high rates of chronic disease.

bananas on your cereal instead of sugar. In time your tastes will change, and you will actually prefer less concentrated sweets.

It doesn't mean that you have to give up your favorite desserts altogether. Use moderation.

Begin by decreasing the frequency of eating sugared foods. Work from "several times daily" to "three times a week." When desserts are served less often, you and your family will begin looking forward to them and enjoy them more.

Another aspect of moderation is learning to be satisfied with smaller portions. Big servings and second helpings are just bad habits. You can learn to enjoy one piece of chocolate candy as much as eating the whole box. And you'll feel better! Half a normal slice of pie or cake, eaten slowly and with pleasure, can be more satisfying than a larger piece bolted down.

Reducing the amount of refined and concentrated sugars in the diet and eating more high-fiber foods, such as whole grains, legumes, vegetables, and fruits, will produce the right kind of sugar highs. These highs will keep you energetic and feeling good all day long.

NOTES

Refined sugars make up some 21 percent of the calories most Americans eat. Much of this sugar is well hidden in food and beverages. To reduce the sugar in your diet, start by substituting naturally sweet foods for sugared snacks.

Reducing the Sugar in Your Diet

Sugar contains no nutrients or fiber. It's high in calories and can crowd more nutritious foods out of your diet.

If sugar has a grip on you, here are three simple tips to help you reduce your dependence without eliminating sweet treats altogether.

1. Indulge Less Frequently

How often do you eat desserts or sweet snacks?

__ 1-4 times/week   __ 1-2 times/day
__ 3-4 times/day   __ more than 4 times/day

If you answered more than once a day, you would benefit from reserving treats for special times.

Reeducate Your Sweet Tooth

A sweet tooth can be reeducated to enjoy less concentrated sweets. Fruit and desserts sweetened with fruit are good alternatives. Try this recipe for a special treat:

Fruit Smoothies

- 2 frozen, ripe bananas
- 1 c pineapple juice
- 3 or 4 soft dates
- 2 c frozen fruit*

Blend dates and pineapple juice until smooth. Add bananas and fruit. Blend until it is the consistency of soft ice cream. Delicious! It also makes a great topping for whole-grain waffles and pancakes.

*Try these kinds:

strawberries	blueberries
peaches	crushed pineapple
orange juice	blackberries

2. Eat Smaller Servings

When you do eat sweets and sugared foods, learn to savor small portions. Eat slowly, and make your portion last. You can train yourself to be satisfied with a smaller serving.

3. Make the Low-Sugar Choice

Choose low-sugar alternatives when shopping. It's not always easy to tell how much sugar a product contains, because sugar can be disguised as fructose, sucrose, corn syrup, and other ingredients. When possible, however, buy products you know are low in sugar.

Your Turn

Think of some ways you can reduce the amount of sugar you are eating. List them below:

_____

_____

_____

_____

Your Challenge

Become more aware of how many sweets and other sugary foods you are eating, by recording it for a day. Then begin to cut back to a healthier level.

The Lowdown on "Wheat" Bread

"Imitation Bread—Stuff of Lies" is what a best-selling author calls today's white bread. "It's a bizarre combination of the least-nutritious part of the wheat grain and a number of artificial chemicals, which can be harmful."

What's wrong with white bread?

Basically, what's wrong is what the milling process does to wheat. A grain of wheat is made up of an outer covering (bran), an embryo (wheat germ), and the endosperm (see graph on next page).

The *bran* contains most of the fiber, generous amounts of vitamins and minerals, and a bit of protein.

The *germ* is a rich source of B and E vitamins, several minerals, and fiber.

The *endosperm*, which makes up roughly four fifths of the whole-wheat kernel, contains mostly starch. It is the only part used in making white flour. Ironically, the nutritious bran and wheat germ, which are removed during the milling process, are sold for animal feed.

The food industry further compounds the nutritional problems by using several artificial chemicals, such as:

- Propylene glycol (antifreeze) to keep bread white.
- Diacetyl tartaric acid (an emulsifier) to save on shortening.
- Calcium sulfate (plaster of Paris) to make it easier to knead large batches of dough.

> "Why spend money on what is not bread, and your labor on what does not satisfy? Listen, listen to me, and eat what is good."
> —Isaiah 55:2

Should we avoid eating white bread?

No bread is all bad. Even the white, fluffy stuff is a high-starch and low-fat food. It's just that some breads are much better than others.

Take fiber, for instance. A slice of white bread contains about a half gram of fiber, while a slice of 100 percent whole-wheat bread contains two grams, and some whole-grain breads contain as much as four grams of fiber per slice. This means you'd need to eat eight slices of white bread to get the fiber of one slice of whole-grain bread.

What about *enriched flour* and *enriched* bread?

During the milling of wheat, some 20 known minerals and vitamins are largely removed. When nutritional deficiency diseases emerged some years back as a result of commercial milling, the industry started an enrichment program. Four of the nutrients were restored—thiamine, riboflavin, niacin, and iron—and the bread was renamed "enriched." However, in most cases, not much was or has been done about the other nutrients lost or reduced in the milling process.

What kind of bread is the most healthful?

Truly healthful bread contains ground-up whole grains, with the bran, germ, and endosperm present. Such breads have double, triple, and in some cases quadruple nutrient value when compared with their refined counterparts.

When combined with fresh fruit, cereals, vegetables, potatoes, and

On any given day, about 75 percent of the population eats white bread or rolls, while only 25 percent eat whole-wheat or rye.

beans, bread makes interesting and satisfying meals and helps maintain good energy levels for long periods.

Look for the substantial-feeling loaves that aren't full of air. Look for 100 percent whole-wheat, stone-ground if possible. Sprouted-wheat breads are also excellent.

Find a reliable bakery. Better yet, make your own bread.

Whole-wheat flour seems to attract weevils!

Whole-grain flours have a healthy balance of starch, protein, natural fats, and fiber besides being loaded with vitamins and minerals. The bugs seem to know this. White flour, on the other hand, is such a nutritional minus that the bugs are too smart to touch it.

Store whole-grain flours in your refrigerator or freezer. Or buy the grains whole and grind them up into flour just before using.

Isn't bread, even whole-wheat bread, fattening?

It isn't the bread that's fattening, but what has been done to it. A slice of whole-wheat bread has 70 calories—no more than an apple. If slathered with peanut butter and jam, the slice can pack close to 300 calories. It's not the raw materials but the overhead

A KERNAL OF WHEAT

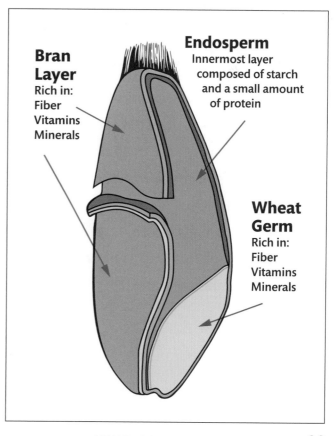

Bran Layer
Rich in:
Fiber
Vitamins
Minerals

Endosperm
Innermost layer composed of starch and a small amount of protein

Wheat Germ
Rich in:
Fiber
Vitamins
Minerals

Look Past the Hype

Because no bread is all bad, the makers of even the least-nutritious loaves capitalize on this. The wrappers boldly proclaim "wholesome goodness," "natural," and "fiber." Names such as Roman Meal, 12-grain, stone-ground wheat, old-fashioned oatmeal, country, rustic, and multigrain sound as though they are overflowing with good stuff. Mostly, they are "overflowing" with white flour—with just a touch of some kinds of whole wheat or other whole grain.

Choices

White Flour, whether in a pretzel or a baguette, is digested rapidly, so it can leave you with almost the same energy shortfall you would get from a candy bar. Coarse, salt-of-the-earth breads, however, provide hours of fuel; that means hours of sustained energy.

Percent Loss of Nutrients When Refining Wheat			
Thiamine (B$_1$)	86	Calcium	50
Riboflavin (B$_2$)	70	Phosphorus	78
Niacin (B$_3$)	80	Copper	75
Iron	84	Magnesium	72
Manganese	71	Biotin	90
Folic Acid	70	Zinc	71
Chromium	87	Fiber	68

that can turn a low-calorie, nutritious, healthful slice of good bread into a caloric disaster.

Bread has traditionally been the backbone of human nutrition. Restoring good bread to its rightful place is a big step toward better health. Next time you shop for bread, go for the real staff of life.

NOTES

Application

During the milling process wheat loses much of its nutrients and fiber. That's why it is important to shop for 100 percent whole-wheat bread. It is better balanced and more nutritious than white bread.

Take a Closer Look

Below are the ingredient lists from three loaves of bread. Which one would you choose for optimum nutrition?

Loaf 1: Whole cracked wheat, unbleached enriched wheat flour (flour, malted barley flour, reduced iron, niacin, thiamine mononitrate, riboflavin), water, honey, raisin syrup, salt, butter, ground raisins, unprocessed miller's bran, partially hydrogenated soybean oil, yeast, wheat gluten, wheat germ, vinegar, lecithin.

Loaf 2: Stone-ground whole-wheat flour, multigrain cereal (rolled oats, rye, cornmeal, sunflower seeds, flaxseeds, wheat germ, soyflour), honey, canola oil, yeast, sea salt, vinegar.

Loaf 3: Enriched bleached flour (barley malt, iron, niacin, thiamine mononitrate, riboflavin) water, corn syrup, soybean oil, yeast, salt, corn flour, whey, soy flour, cornstarch, nonfat milk, fungal enzymes, ammonia chloride, calcium sulfate, potassium bromate, mono- and diglycerides.

Which loaf did you pick?

Did You Make the Best Choice?

Loaf 1: This loaf isn't bad. The first ingredient is whole cracked wheat. Its second ingredient, however, is enriched wheat flour—white flour. It has diminished amounts of most vitamins, minerals, and fiber of whole-grain flour.

Loaf 2: This is the best choice. Its first ingredient is whole-wheat flour. Its second ingredient is seven-grain cereal, which adds the nutrition of a variety of whole grains to the loaf. This loaf feels heavier and more dense than the others.

Loaf 3: This is a loaf of spongy white bread. It contains lesser amounts of vitamins, minerals, and fiber. It's not the best choice for the health-conscious shopper.

Your Challenge

Look for whole-grain breads when you shop. Read the labels carefully, and don't be misled by packaging that tries to pass off the "stuff of lies" as the "staff of life."

NOTES

Delicious Fruit Spread

Try these delicious toppings on whole-grain toast.

Strawberry Spread
1 c strawberries
1 c mashed, ripe banana

Blend ingredients in a blender until smooth. Pour in saucepan, thicken with some cornstarch. Bring to a rapid boil.

Can We Eat Too Much?

*Protein originates
in plant food.*

A sk any 14-year-old boy whether he would rather grow bigger faster or live longer, and he would probably choose growing bigger faster.

Is that a relevant question?

Yes, because in the 1930s studies on laboratory animals began to turn up evidence that high-protein diets accelerated growth rate and maturation, but shortened the life span.

In animals, maybe. But everyone knows that humans need plenty of protein!

Back in 1880 a German scientist, Justus von Liebig, determined that muscles were made of protein. His protegé, Karl Voit, watching coal miners, calculated that these strong, muscular men ate around 120 grams of protein a day. He concluded from this observation that this was the ideal amount to eat. Ever since, getting enough protein has been an obsession that persists to this day.

How much protein do we really need?

Modern scientific studies show that adults actually need only about 30 grams of protein a day. The human body very efficiently harvests and recycles its own protein. The only protein losses that need to be replaced are those that the body cannot retrieve, such as hair, fingernails and toenails, and skin.

So we need only 30 grams of protein a day?

The National Academy of Sciences sets the American Recommended Daily Intake (RDI) for vitamins, minerals, and certain foods. The RDI for protein has been set at 0.35 grams per pound of ideal body weight. This is more than the 30 grams/day minimum requirement. It works out to 60 grams for a 170-pound man and 45 grams for a 128-pound woman. Even so, the average Westerner continues to eat between 100 to 130 grams of protein a day (see graph on next page).

Is that a problem?

- Most of the protein eaten by Westerners comes from animal sources and is loaded with cholesterol and fat. Because fat is well hidden, many people don't realize that meats, sausages, and dairy products average from 50 to 88 percent of their calories as fat calories. Excess fat and cholesterol, and especially saturated fat, are known for their atherosclerosis-promoting effects, which lead to narrowing, hardening, and increase of plaque in vital oxygen-carrying arteries. This process accelerates aging and shortens life.
- A high-protein diet cuts endurance. Athletes now load up on complex carbohydrates rather than on protein.
- Excess protein places added burdens on the kidneys. Kidney disease is increasingly common in Western culture.
- High animal-protein diets are associated with osteoporosis. The processing of excess protein by the kidneys requires calcium, much of which is leached from the bones.
- From 1850 to 2010 the average age of sexual maturity for American teenage girls declined from 16.3 years to 11.7 years. The meat-centered diet is implicated.
- High intake of animal protein promotes the growth of several cancers.

Don't children need extra protein?

Yes, they do, especially during periods of rapid growth. The RDI of 0.35 grams per pound of ideal body weight works out to 17 grams of protein a day for a 50-pound child—a little more than half an ounce. Since children in Western cultures eat the same high-protein diets that adults do, there is very little concern for not getting enough protein!

The problem may well be on the other side of the question. Accumulating evidence suggests that children eating high-fat and -protein diets tend to grow bigger and develop faster. Are they paying the price of a shortened life?

What about the amino acid arguments?

Proteins are made of some 20 amino acids. While the body can manufacture 12 of these building

PROTEIN CONTENT IN FOOD PRODUCTS

U.S. Diet	Grams	Optimal Diet	Grams
3-Egg Ham and Cheese Omelet	46	Cooked Cereal	9
Hash browns	3	With Milk and 1/2 Banana	11
Toast (2) With Butter, Jelly	5	Toast (2) With 1/2 Banana	4
Orange Juice	1	Fruit (Orange)	1
Breakfast Total	**55**	**Breakfast Total**	**25**
Big Mac	26	Pita Bread (3) Stuffed With Tomatoes, Sprouts, Cucumbers	8
French Fries	3	Three-Bean Salad	10
Milk Shake	11	Split-Pea Soup With Barley	12
Lunch Total	**40**	**Lunch Total**	**30**
Fried Chicken (Basket)	48	Spaghetti With Tomato Sauce	10
Mixed Salad, Dressing	4	Tossed Salad	4
Baked Potato, Sour Cream	9	Broccoli Flowerets	5
Peas	5	Bread (2) With Garbanzo Spread	10
Milk	9	Baked Apple With Walnuts	1
Dinner Total	**75**	**Dinner Total**	**30**
Total Grams of Protein	**170**	**Total Grams of Protein**	**85**

Urea is produced in the processing of protein by the liver.

In excess, urea acts as a diuretic. A high protein intake may require up to seven times as much water to wash out the waste products from the kidneys.

PROTEIN

FOOD COMPOSITION (in percent of calories)

	Protein	Fat	Carbohydrate
Meat	**32%**	**68%**	**0%**
Beef	25	75	0
Pork	25	75	0
Chicken	45	55	0
Dairy	**29%**	**41%**	**30%**
Milk, whole	21	48	31
Milk, skim	40	3	57
Cheese	25	73	2
Nuts	**9%**	**87%**	**4%**
Almonds	12	82	6
Pecans	5	93	2
Walnuts	9	88	3
Legumes	**29%**	**12%**	**59%**
Soybeans	33	30	37
Pinto beans	26	3	71
Lentils	29	3	68
Grains	**13%**	**8%**	**79%**
Rice, brown	8	4	88
Oatmeal	14	16	70
Wheat, whole	16	5	79
Vegetables	**14%**	**4%**	**82%**
Cabbage	22	7	71
Carrots	10	4	86
Potatoes	11	1	88
Fruits	**6%**	**3%**	**91%**
Bananas	5	2	93
Peaches	6	2	92
Oranges	8	4	88

blocks, eight amino acids have been demonstrated to be essential for adults. They have to be provided by the diet. People used to believe that they had to eat meat and dairy products in order to supply these "essential" amino acids. The fact that these foods are high in fat and cholesterol, lack fiber, and have detrimental effects on health was, for many years, overlooked or considered irrelevant.

Now we know that these amino acids are easily available from a random selection of plant foods, *augmented by the amino acid pool of the body*. This is shown in dietary patterns around the world. The staple food in Caribbean countries is black beans and rice. Certain amino acids low in rice are found in the beans, and vice versa. The same is true for the corn tortillas and pinto beans of the Mexicans, and the rice and soybeans relied upon by the Chinese.

The Western world is taking a fresh look at plant foods. They are low in fat, high in fiber, free of cholesterol, full of nutrients, and have plenty of protein. The protein content of many vegetables exceeds 20 percent of total calories, while whole grains average about 12 percent and most legumes average 30 percent.

Progressive nutritionists advise getting 10 percent of daily calories as protein. Even on a total vegetarian diet, getting this much protein is obviously no problem. In fact, when enough calories are available from a variety of unrefined plant foods, it's impossible to create a protein deficiency.

It's time to bury the myth and catch up with the times. With protein, as with much else in life, too much of a good thing is a bad thing.

NOTES

Most North Americans eat twice as much protein as is recommended. This excess has been linked to kidney disease, gout, and osteoporosis. Large quantities of meat and dairy products are not needed—vegetable sources are ideal to provide your body with all the protein it needs.

The Protein Myth

What kind of foods come to mind when you hear the word protein? Beef? Pork? Chicken? Eggs? Advertisers spend millions each year making certain we feel these foods are indispensable for good health.

The fact is—animal products are not needed in the human diet. People may choose to eat them for reasons of flavor, habit, and convenience, but nobody should feel they must eat them to get enough protein or sufficient nutrients.

Plant Protein

All the protein you need is available from plant sources. Traditional "high-protein" foods are largely very high in fat, high in cholesterol, and they lack fiber. Plant foods, however, are naturally low in fat, high in fiber, and they are devoid of cholesterol. If you eat a variety of grains, legumes, and vegetables, your diet will never lack the protein your body needs for optimal performance and well-being.

What Are You Eating?

Look at the table in this chapter. Which foods don't you usually eat? List them below.

_____

_____

_____

_____

Your Challenge

Stretch the boundaries of your diet by sampling some of the foods you have listed. Experiment with the wide variety of tastes and textures available.

Easy Zucchini

6 small zucchinis
3 c tomato juice
1/4 tsp thyme
1/2 tsp *Mrs. Dash*

Slice zucchini into 1/4-inch-thick slices. Place them into baking dish with other ingredients. Cover and bake at 375°F for 20 minutes.

NOTES

_____

_____

_____

_____

_____

_____

_____

Who Needs It?

Humans are the only mammals who drink milk after the weaning period.

Milk is the perfect food—for babies. But make no mistake: breast is best for each of the 4,300 species of mammals on earth, because each mammal's milk is precisely designed and balanced for its own young. That's why cow's milk is best—but only for baby calves.

Are you saying that cow's milk shouldn't be given to human babies?

That's right! The American College of Pediatrics strongly urges that cow's milk should not be given to children until they are at least 1 year of age. There are many good reasons for this. A few examples:

- Allergies and asthma have reached epidemic proportions in the United States. Infants not exposed to cow's milk develop far fewer allergies; they also experience much less colic, eczema, and nasal and bronchial congestion.
- Babies need the antibodies (immunities) found in breast milk to protect them from infectious diseases. Scientists have discovered more than 90 elements in mother's milk, with concentrations changing over time to accommodate the needs of the developing child.
- Breast milk is sterile, unlike cow's milk, which is regularly contaminated.
- The protein in cow's milk is suspected of being able to trigger diabetes in infants.
- Despite antibiotics, infants who have been fed formula or cow's milk are 70 percent more likely to develop diarrhea and ear infections when compared to babies exclusively breast-fed.

After the first year, then, isn't milk a healthful food?

Not really. For years we've been led to believe that milk is indispensable for sound health. The average Westerner, however, eats too much fat, too much cholesterol, too much protein, and not enough fiber. Whole milk, when calculated in percent of total calories, is just about 50 percent fat (much of it saturated) and 20 percent protein. It contains cholesterol and has no dietary fiber. In many ways it resembles the composition of meat. Drinking milk puts added burdens on an already-overloaded metabolic system.

How about low-fat milk? Doesn't that solve most of the problems?

Low-fat milk is an improvement over whole milk, but not as great as it seems. For one reason, it does not solve the lactose intolerance/lactose deficiency problem.

For another, it still contains too much fat. The 2 percent fat in low-fat milk is calculated from the weight of the milk, not from its calories. By *weight,* this milk is 87 percent water and 2 percent fat. By *calories,* however, it is a 30 percent fat food.

Nonfat milk (skim milk) is the best choice for those who can tolerate or wish to drink milk. Nonfat milk has no fat, and is virtually cholesterol-free, yet retains its other nutrients.

But by removing the fat, it increases the amount of protein, and with that the amount of casein, a prominent milk protein. This protein has been implicated with significantly promoting the growth

WHOLE MILK FAT CONTENT

Whole milk (2 glasses) = 3.7% fat by weight	
Total Calories	300
Grams of fat	16.8
Calories of fat (16.8 gm fat x 9 cal/gm)	150
150 of the 300 calories in milk come from fat.	
Whole milk = 50% fat by calories	

of tumors in animal experiments. Increasing or decreasing the amount of casein in the rat chow would either turn on or off the tumor growth.

The Federal Trade Commission (FTC) took the American Dairy Association to task for engaging in FALSE ADVERTISING by using the slogan "Everybody Needs Milk."

How about calcium? Isn't milk needed for its calcium content to prevent osteoporosis?

It's true that milk is high in calcium, but that isn't the whole story. The dairy industry capitalizes on the concern about osteoporosis and pushes its products beyond all reason. For example:

- International studies have shown that a high calcium intake does not necessarily insure or protect against osteoporosis. Traditionally, Eskimos have eaten in excess of 2,000 milligrams of calcium per day, yet osteoporosis is rampant in that population. On the other hand, osteoporosis is hard to find among millions of Bantus in central Africa even though they consume less than 400 milligrams of calcium a day.
- Generally speaking, and paradoxically, cultures with the high-

est dairy consumption have the highest rates of osteoporosis, a disease rarely found in non-milk-drinking countries. While milk carries plenty of calcium, its relatively high protein content, when added to the large amounts of protein consumed in the form of meat, fowl, and fish, actually leaches calcium from the bones as it is being metabolized (see pages 56-59).

- Actually only 25 to 30 percent of the calcium in milk is absorbed by the human body.

Are those the main problems with milk?

Unfortunately there are more.

- The incidence of coronary heart disease in North America is much higher than in non-dairy-using cultures. Whole milk and cheese, with their saturated fat and cholesterol, contribute to heart disease.
- Certain proteins raise blood cholesterol levels, and casein, a common milk protein, is one of the worst.
- Each animal's milk is designed to fit the growth rates of its own young. Human babies develop very slowly, and the composition of human milk reflects that difference. Animal milks may contribute to the earlier maturation noted in many of today's children.
- After weaning, many humans exhibit lactose intolerance / lac-

Mom's Own Milk

Infantile colic symptoms disappeared in one third of breast-fed infants when the mother stopped drinking cow's milk.

Everybody Knows That Milk Is for Babies...

But shouldn't adults be leaning toward weaning?

tose deficiency. This refers to the inability to digest and metabolize lactose, a sugar found in milk. It is related to a lack of the enzyme lactase in the digestive system required to break down lactose. It results in symptoms including abdominal pain and bloating, flatuleuce (gas). Lack for decreased lactate activity differs with ethnic groups. Here is the distribution of lactose intolerance / lactose deficiency for ethinic groups in North America.

Lactose Intolerance by Ethnic Groups (US)	
North European Descent	5%
Silicilian Descent	up to 70%
Afro-American	up to 80%
Asian Descent	100%
American Indian	up to 100%

- Several studies have implicated milk and other dairy products as probable contributors to breast cancer. In men who regularly drank more than two glasses of milk per day, prostate cancer risk jumped 400 percent (see pages 48-51).
- Infectious agents can be effectively transmitted through milk, ice cream, and cheese. Hormones, antibiotic residues, viruses, pesticides, industrial chemicals, and other contaminants can also find their way into milk.
- Just as some bacteria can survive the pasteurization process, so do many viruses, including certain leukemia and sarcoma viruses. Another worry is that prions, which come from cattle with mad cow disease, may taint milk. Not even boiling will inactivate these disease-causing prions.

Are you implying that adult humans don't need milk?

Many people live their whole lives in good health without drinking milk or using other dairy products. If used at all, milk should be consumed—preferably in nonfat form—in small quantities, such as in cooking or baking.

Many concerned people are choosing other sources of calcium (grains, legumes, vegetable greens).

Moreover, an abundance of milk-like products is now available that are suitable substitutes for animal milks. Most food stores have liberal supplies of various kinds of soy milk products, or "milks" made from rice, oatmeal, potato, and almond, that are all calcium fortified.

All the nutrients we need for maximum health can be obtained without resorting to dairy foods. And there is a bonus: we can also avoid a host of "problems" by shunning these harmful substances.

Remember—every creature's milk is a health food—but only for its own offspring. Milk is the perfect food—for baby calves.

NOTES

Milk is a concentrated protein and as cheese a very high-fat food. If used at all, it should be used sparingly in nonfat form. Many types of soy or tofu milks are now commercially available. They make excellent milk substitutes.

The Optimal Diet

Research on nutrition has clearly demonstrated a unitary dietary principle in dealing with our Western killer diseases. There isn't one diet for treating heart disease, and another for overweight, and yet another for hypertension and diabetes.

Instead, there is one optimal diet consisting of a wide variety of plant foods, freely eaten "as grown," prepared with sparing use of fats, oils, sugars, and salt, and almost devoid of refined or processed foods. If animal products are eaten, they are best used more like a seasoning, more for the flavor and not as the focus of the meal.

Take a look at how the *Western diet* compares with *the Optimal diet* (see graph).

Your Challenge

Pick up some samples of milk substitutes and embark on a new habit of dairy-free living. And observe the impact on your health.

Current U.S. Public Health Service regulations state that milk, after pasteurization, should contain no more than 20,000 bacteria/milliliter of milk and no more than 10 coliform bacteria/milliliter. This means that a glass of milk with up to 5 million bacteria is still acceptable. It also means that 2,500 of these coliform bacteria are allowed per eight ounces of milk.

COMPARISON OF DIETS *(per day)*

Food Item/Day	Western Diet	Optimal Diet
Fats and Oils	80-120 gm	under 45 gm
Complex Carbohydrates	20-25%	65-75%
Protein	80-120gm	50-60 gm
Refined Sugar	40 tsp	under 10 tsp
Cholesterol	400 mg	under 50 mg
Salt	10 gm	under 5 gm
Fiber	10 gm	30 gm plus
Water (fluids)	minimal	8 glasses plus

COMPARISON OF MILKS OF DIFFERENT SPECIES

Milk of	Mean values for protein content*	Time required to double birth weight
Human	1.2%	180 days
Mare	2.4%	60 days
Cow	3.3%	47 days
Goat	4.1%	19 days
Dog	7.1%	8 days
Cat	9.5%	7 days

*by weight

NOTES

Looking for the Real Food

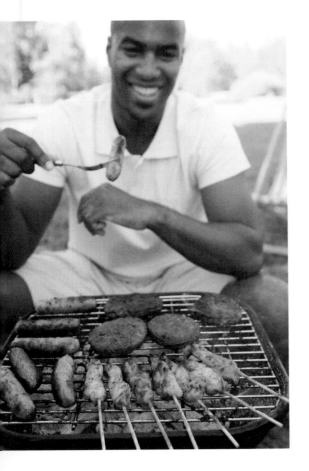

> "A total vegetarian diet can prevent up to 97 percent of our heart attacks."
>
> —*Journal of the American Medical Association*

R eal food! In fact, real food for real people! What an attractive thought! What an exciting promise!

Real food? Are you talking about those old commercials?

The commercials may be history, but the sound bite is brilliant. The real food turns out to be beef—and a beautiful girl croons that she's not sure she wants to know anyone who doesn't eat it. A macho actor complains that vegetables fall off his shish kebab. An authoritative voice informs us that three ounces of the new, leaner cuts of beef contain no more cholesterol than is found in three ounces of chicken.

What that voice didn't tell you is that lean beef, while comparable to chicken in cholesterol content, contains three to six times more dangerous, cholesterol-raising saturated fat. Besides, who eats three-ounce portions? The average hamburger weighs close to five ounces, and an average-size steak weighs in at six ounces.

But isn't meat an important source of protein?

Meat is a nutritious source of protein, but it carries along a number of problems:

For one thing, most people overestimate their protein needs. The Recommended Daily Intake (RDI) for protein is a generously adequate 45 to 60 grams. Most Westerners, however, consume twice this much. These excessive amounts of protein are hard on the kidneys, promote gout, and cause calcium to be leached from the bones.

An even bigger problem is the hefty dose of fat (mostly saturated) and cholesterol. Scientific research has overwhelmingly implicated a rich diet as the major culprit in today's chronic killer diseases. And the rich foods that are doing us in are mostly animal products, such as meat, fowl, eggs, and dairy products.

The trouble is, while the human body is able to nourish itself on animal foods, it lacks protection against large amounts of fat and cholesterol. Excessive fat and cholesterol stack up in the bloodstream and begin attaching themselves to the linings of blood vessels. Gradually, over time, plaques form, arterial walls thicken and harden, arterial lumens narrow, and atherosclerosis has established itself.

As a result, blood supplies to vital organs diminish or get cut off, and the stage is set for many of today's killer diseases, such as heart disease, hypertension, stroke, arthritis, diabetes, and several types of adult cancer.

Americans have always eaten meat. Why all these problems now?

- Let's look at the turn of the century. We didn't have many of these atherosclerosis-related diseases because in 1900 we didn't eat meat two or three times a day as we do now. Some 70 percent of our protein then came from plant foods. Today we get 70 percent of our protein from animal sources loaded with saturated fat and cholesterol.
- We also raised our animals differently then. Chickens scratched in barnyards and pigs loafed around in mudholes. These idyllic, happy farms, however, have been replaced by today's factory farms. The greatest possible number of animals are raised in the smallest possible space at the lowest possible cost. Most food animals today are raised on feedlots or contained in cages, with practically no exercise. The meat from these animals may

contain up to twice as much fat as the meat from range-fed and free farm animals.
- Animals ingest and store chemicals in their bodies from the fertilizers and pesticides used on their food. Hormones, antibiotics, and other chemicals also often are routinely administered

USDA studies show that more than one third of broiler chicken carcasses on the market are contaminated with illness-causing bacteria.

to animals in intensive confinement systems to mask stress and disease and to speed growth. Residues of these contaminants find their way into the food chain.

To those willing to look at the evidence, the bulk of the scientific literature implicates a rich diet as the major culprit in today's health problems. Those culprits are mainly animal foods.

The message, however, is slowly getting through: Americans today consume less beef, eggs, whole milk, and butter than they did 10 years ago. But, regrettably, they don't replace them with products of the plant kingdom, but with chicken, turkey, lobsters, shrimp, and cheese.

Are you suggesting that a meatless lifestyle is better?

Billions of people around the world are getting along just fine on plant protein diets. Here are some of the advantages:

Health Advantages

People who don't eat animal products have:
- Fewer heart attacks and strokes
- Fewer weight problems
  - Lower cholesterol
  - Lower blood pressure
  - Less diabetes
  - Fewer hemorrhoids, less diverticular disease, and good regularity
  - Less cancer of the breast, prostate, and colon
  - Stronger bones, less osteoporosis
  - Fewer stones of the kidney and gallbladder, and less kidney disease, and gouty arthritis

And they live longer!

In addition, such a diet is fun, rewarding, and cost-effective.

Environmental Advantages

Animal agriculture is the single most environmentally destructive industry in the world. Switching to a meatless diet would—
- Conserve water: Some 25 gallons are needed to produce one pound of wheat, whereas 2,500 gallons are needed to produce one pound of beef.
- Protect rain forests: Producing a single pound of hamburger in Costa Rica involves the destruction of 55 square feet of rain forest to grow the needed animal food.
- Preserve topsoil: Every year 5 billion tons of topsoil are lost in the U.S. largely because of overgraz-

Summary

- Raising animals for food wastes foodstuffs that should be used to feed the world's hungry people and depletes drastically our irreplaceable food production resources, such as topsoil and groundwater.
- Raising animals for food devastates forests and other wildlife habitats and dumps more pollutants into our lakes and streams than all other human activities combined.
- Raising animals for food on today's factory farms involves the confinement, crowding, deprivation, mutilation, and other gross abuse and slaughter of nearly 9 billion feeling, innocent animals.
- Consumption of animal fat and meat has been linked conclusively with a high incidence of heart disease, stroke, cancer, and other chronic diseases that cripple and kill 1.5 million Americans each year.
- 1 million animals are killed in America *every hour!*

ing of livestock and unsustainable methods of growing animal feed.

- Save trees: Forests are cleared to raise crops for animal feed. Each meat eater who switches will save an acre of trees per year.
- Keep water clean: Every year American feedlot operations alone produce 1 billion tons of animal wastes—a significant source of water pollution.

World Food Supplies Advantages

About 85 percent of American-grown grain is fed to animals. If Americans would cut their meat consumption in half, the land, water, grain, and soybeans saved could feed the entire developing world.

That's pretty impressive!

The evidence against meat and other animal products is stacking up as nutritional research confirms that a diet built around whole plant food is not only adequate but superior.

Humans don't have the instinct to kill.

We are more apt to salivate over a bunch of chilled grapes than a piece of raw meat. It's comforting to know that a diet of fruit, vegetables, legumes, grains and some nuts is perfectly suited to our needs—anatomically, physiologically, and instinctively.

It's not easy, however, to examine our lifelong eating habits and to find them wanting. But the wise among us will examine. And the wise among us will not look to the slaughterhouses or to the factories to find real food. The wise among us will find the real food in the gardens and farms of our land.

NOTES

_____

_____

_____

_____

_____

_____

_____

Application

The evidence keeps mounting that a diet built around whole plant foods is superior to a meat-based diet. Meat is high in fat and cholesterol. It also lacks the fiber found in foods "as grown." In populations around the world, vegetarians have better health, are thinner, and live longer.

Kicking the Meat Habit

Many, who have made meat and dairy products the center of their meals, feel at a loss when trying to plan a meatless menu. For a while their meals seem incomplete without flesh foods.

You can satisfy your appetite on a meat-free diet. It may take a while to adjust. But eventually this way of eating becomes acceptable, and then preferable. Here is a sample menu to get you started planning delicious meat-free meals:

Sample Menu
Breakfast:
- Cooked cereal (seven-grain cereal) or cold cereal (Shredded Wheat, Nutrigrain) with skim milk or a milk substitute, and half of a banana or other fresh fruit sliced on top.
- Citrus fruit: orange or grapefruit—peel and eat the whole fruit.
- Three slices of whole-wheat toast with "mashed" banana topped with pineapple ring or slice of kiwi.
- Herbal tea.

Lunch:
- Two whole-wheat pita (pocket) breads stuffed with lettuce, sprouts, cucumbers, tomatoes, radishes and some low-fat cottage cheese or its tofu equivalent.
- Split-pea soup with pearl barley or rice.
- Fresh fruit such as papaya, pear, apple, or mango.

Dinner:
- Whole-wheat spaghetti and tomato sauce.
- Tossed salad with a low-calorie Italian dressing.
- Slice of whole-grain bread
- For dessert: baked apple with date and a walnut.

Food Selection

Develop your own one-day menu. Use the guidelines provided. Enjoy!

Selection Suggestions
Optimal Foods
Fruit: all fresh fruit (avocados and olives sparingly).

Vegetables: vegetables, greens, herbs, and squash.

Legumes: all beans, peas, lentils, garbanzos.

Tubers: potatoes, yams, sweet potatoes.

Grains: all whole grains, bread, pasta.

Nuts: use sparingly.

Optional Foods *(if you feel you must use them)*
Dairy: nonfat milk, plain yogurt, skim milk cheeses, buttermilk, and low-fat cottage cheese – all in moderation.

Eggs: whites only—or replace with *Ener-G* powder for binding.

Meats: small amounts, if you insist. Skinless fowl, fish fillet, lean beef.

Your Challenge

As you are planning a more natural dietary program, build your meals around the food categories listed above.

The Bad News Is Really Good News

An insidious villain is at work in our country quietly disabling and killing more Americans each year than all the wars in this century. The villain? The fat in our food!

Are you saying that eating fat can kill us?

The excess fat in food is being singled out as the most damaging component of the Western diet. That deadly duo—the high-fat, low-fiber diet—is now linked to such diverse problems as coronary artery (heart) disease; obesity; gallstones; appendicitis; cancers of the colon, breast, and prostate; strokes; constipation; and diverticulitis, to name a few. And the list continues to grow.

Don't we need fat to be healthy?

Fat is a vital part of every living cell. Fat is also the body's backup fuel system. We could not be optimally healthy without fat in our diets.

Problems occur when we eat too much fat and of the wrong kind. We understand that a car runs best with its specified fuel. We might get a car to run on kerosene, but it would be disastrous to its engine. Improper fuel damages the body motor also, though it's not as readily seen because a healthy body has great reserves. Up to 80 percent of the liver and kidneys can be destroyed before the organs go into failure. By the time the first anginal pain or heart attack is experienced, the diameter of coronary arteries in important locations may already be reduced by 80 percent or more.

Get the "Fat Tooth" Pulled!

We eat two to three times more fat, oil, and grease than appears ideal. The average North American diet contains 80 to 120 grams of fat (about 35-40 percent of total calories). Many researchers feel it ought to be under 45 grams (about 10-20 percent of total calories).

How does fat damage the body?

An excessive amount of fat in the diet sets up conditions for the development of atherosclerosis—a hardening and narrowing of vital arteries that supply nutrients and oxygen to the body. Excess fat makes the blood thick and sticky, slowing circulation and causing red blood cells to adhere to each other in bunches. These clumped blood cells cannot carry their full load of oxygen, and they are unable to navigate tiny capillaries. Deprived of oxygen and nutrients, body cells become susceptible to injury, disease, and death.

Most high-fat foods are loaded with cholesterol, which injures the linings of arteries. The body responds by sealing off these damaged spots with extra cells. In the presence of excess fat and cholesterol more and more "band-aids" are added, one on top of the other, until plaques are formed. When plaques grow large enough to narrow and obstruct coronary arteries, heart attacks occur. When it happens in arteries feeding the brain, strokes occur.

Some of the by-products of fat digestion appear to be involved in the promotion of certain cancers. These substances often cause irritation and inflammation of bowel walls, and may be a factor in colitis and colon cancer. When adequate fiber is present, however, feces move along quickly, leaving less time for toxic carcinogens to act on bowel walls.

On another front, excess fat in the bloodstream is one of the factors that depresses immune cell production.

High-fat diets have been shown to impair the efficiency of the body's insulin mechanism, which may lead to diabetes.

Moreover, the amount of saturated fat in the diet, along with the intake of trans fats (hydrogenated) powerfully affect blood cholesterol levels.

What can we do to protect ourselves?

It's crucial that we cut down on the fat in our diets. Butter, margarine, shortening, and cooking and salad oils are nearly 100 percent fat. Meats, cheeses, eggs, and whole milk average 50 to 80 percent of calories as fat.

Furthermore, we need a big increase in fiber intake. Fruits, vegetables, whole grains, and legumes are gaining in popularity. Because these plant foods are high in fiber, low in fat, and free of cholesterol, they are the ideal way to go.

The rich Western diet, bloated with fat, is slowly killing us. We know now that the situation can be turned around by replacing most of the fat calories we eat with unrefined plant foods.

WHERE IS THE FAT?

Foods	Percent Fat Calories	Total Calories Per Cup (8 oz.)
Visible Fats		
Butter, Margarine, Shortening, Lard	100	1,900
Invisible Fats		
Peanut Butter	80	1,500
Nuts	75-92	800
Pork, Beef	65-80	500-800
Double Beef Whopper (Burger King)	60	970
Whole Milk	50	160
Ice Cream	70-80	350
Processed Cheese	60-85	450
Cream Cheese	90	850

Beware!

Of meats and cheeses—

They are largely very calorie-dense foods (fattening), and they have no fiber.

Of trans fats—

Formed when oils are partially hydrogenated to make them spreadable (such as margarine and shortening). These fats raise blood cholesterol levels as much as saturated fat, if not more!

Of saturated fats—

They raise cholesterol levels in the blood, increasing the risk of heart disease and colon and prostate cancer. So keep meat, cheese, pizza, ice cream, whole milk, butter, and most pies, cakes, and pastries in the doghouse.

Of fat-free foods—

Many people feel safe in eating large amounts—but these foods may still be high in calories, especially from sugar.

The good news is that a diet balanced in this manner will prevent many Western-type diseases and help reverse coronary heart disease and most adult diabetes. And there is more. You will enjoy better health and feel more energetic. You can also eat a higher volume of food and lose weight, too!

Design of red blood cell (RBC) maximizes surface area and minimizes volume. Oxygen is carried on the RBC surfaces, which become greatly reduced when RBCs clump in response to a high-fat diet.

More than 50 percent of cancers in the Westernized countries are directly related to overnutrition, particularly the high intake of fat and animal protein of animal origin. To cut the risk of cancer, heart disease, and stroke, people need to eat more protective fruits and vegetables, and much less fat and protein coming from animal sources.

Excess fat in foods is probably the most damaging component of the rich Western diet. Reducing the amount of fat we eat is essential. Butter, margarine, cooking and salad oils, meats, cheeses, eggs, and whole milk all must be limited.

The Old Four Food Groups

In 1956 the U. S. Department of Agriculture developed the Four Food Groups:

1. meats, poultry, fish, eggs, and nuts
2. dairy products (milk and cheese)
3. grains
4. fruits and vegetables

Since then we've discovered a lot about nutrition. One of the things we've learned is that the emphasis on meat and dairy products made the Four Food Groups high in fat, protein, and cholesterol, and low in fiber. Study after study has linked this diet to increased rates of cancer, heart disease, obesity, and diabetes. Clearly a big change is needed: Enter the New Four Food Groups.

Slimming Your Salad Down

One of the best places to cut the fat is on your salad. Too many people take nutritious greens and turn them into a high-fat nightmare by adding thick, oily dressings. Restaurants are notorious for this. At most of them you don't get a little dressing to go with your salad—you get a little salad to go with your dressing.

Next time your waiter hands you a menu, order your salad with a low-calorie dressing on the side. Better yet, ask for lemon wedges and squeeze the juice on yourself. It's a good low-calorie, no-fat alternative.

Your List

Below are the categories from the New Four Food Groups. Under each heading, list foods from that category that you currently eat or would like to try. Chances are you will find that you already eat many foods from the *New Four Food Groups*.

Whole Grains

_____

_____

Vegetables

_____

_____

Fruits

_____

_____

Legumes

_____

_____

Your Challenge

Make the New Four Food Groups the foundation of your diet by eating more of the foods you listed above.

THE NEW FOUR FOOD GROUPS

Recommended by the Physicians' Committee for Responsible Medicine

Food Group	Servings per Day	Serving Size
Whole Grains	five or more	1/2 cup of hot cereal; 1 ounce dry cereal; one slice bread
Vegetables	three or more	one cup raw; 1/2 cup cooked
Legumes	two to three	1/2 cup cooked beans, 4 ounces tofu
Fruits	three or more	one or two medium pieces of fruit; 1/2 cup cooked or 1/4 cup dried fruit

You Need It, But...

Animal products are the largest source of fat in the diet and the only source of cholesterol.

What can turn a normal, needed, healthful substance into a dangerous killer? How can something that makes sex hormones, helps build strong bones, and balances the body's stress response also choke off oxygen and damage vital organs and tissues?

Cholesterol is both hero and villain. While we cannot live without it, in excessive amounts it can kill us.

The blood cholesterol level is the single most important factor in determining a person's risk for heart disease, the nation's number one killer. For instance, a person with a total blood cholesterol level of 260 mg% (6.7 mmol/L) is four times more likely to have a fatal heart attack than is a person with a cholesterol of less than 220 mg% (5.6 mmol/L). And 220 is far from ideal! Every 10 percent rise in blood cholesterol is accompanied by a 30 percent rise in heart attack risk.

Doesn't heredity determine cholesterol level?

Very few people have genetic cholesterol disorders. The vast majority of blood cholesterol levels are determined by dietary factors. Depending on what we eat, cholesterol levels can go up or down substantially, even within a couple weeks.

How does high cholesterol cause heart attacks?

It does it by gradually plugging up the vital heart-nourishing arteries through a process called atherosclerosis.

Most heart attacks are related to plaques, which are made up mostly of cholesterol, fat, and calcium. Plaques are like tire patches. They are the body's response to damaged areas in arterial walls that may be caused by free radicals, especially those found in oxidized cholesterol. The body responds to the irritation by adding more and more "patches" to protect the area, causing the plaque to slowly enlarge. But in doing so it also chokes off the blood flow and may eventually obstruct the artery completely.

When blood cholesterol levels are under 150 mg% (3.8 mmol/L), initial arterial damage usually heals quickly and the scars shrink. But when cholesterol levels edge past 180 (4.6 mmol/L), LDL cholesterol particles begins to attach itself to the vessel walls, causing atherosclerosis (plaque formation, arterial wall thickening and hardening, and arterial narrowing).

Massive studies of world populations have documented the fact that blood cholesterol levels are the most dependable predictor of arterial obstructions resulting from plaque formation. Research on migrant groups of people confirms that this is not so much a disease of genetics as of lifestyle. When people who have been protected by a simple diet move into a Westernized culture with its dietary excesses, their blood cholesterol levels go up, and soon they begin developing the same arterial diseases as Westerners.

But doesn't the body need cholesterol?

Yes, but we don't have to eat it. The liver manufactures all the cholesterol the body needs. But most Westerners eat an additional 400

LIPID LEVELS AND CORONARY RISK

Risk	Total Cholesterol		LDL Cholesterol	
	(mg%)	(mmol/L)	(mg%)	(mmol/L)
Ideal	≤150	≤ 4.0	< 90	< 2.3
Elevated	161-180	4.1-4.6	90-110	< 2.3-2.8
High	181-220	4.7-5.6	111-150	2.9-3.8
Very High	221-260	5.7-6.6	151-190	3.9-4.8
Dangerous	> 260	> 6.6	> 190	> 4.8

milligrams of cholesterol a day. It's this extra dietary cholesterol that causes a considerable part of the problem.

What foods contain cholesterol?

Cholesterol is found only in animal foods. Plant foods do not contain cholesterol. It's as simple as that.

What is a safe blood cholesterol level?

Many heart researchers suggest that cholesterol levels under 150 mg% (3.8 mmol/L) will protect people from atherosclerosis.

Aren't there several kinds of cholesterol in the blood?

Cholesterol never travels alone—in the blood it has different carriers. The heaviest carrier is HDL (high-density lipoprotein), known as the "healthy" cholesterol. HDL is protective in that it removes cholesterol from arteries and takes it to the liver. In the presence of high LDL (low-density lipoprotein), the higher the HDL, the greater the protection.

A lighter cholesterol carrier, the LDL, is the "lethal" one. LDL basically determines the rate at which cholesterol is deposited on artery walls. To be safe, LDL cholesterol should be under 90 mg% (2.3 mmol/L).

A simple way to estimate heart attack risk is to divide the LDL by the HDL. Ideally it should be under 2.0.

While there are several kinds of cholesterol carriers, these two—the HDL and LDL—are the most important ones.

Would you explain "oxidized" cholesterol?

When cholesterol is exposed to air, it can become oxidized by combining with oxygen. Even a small amount of this substance can be quite damaging to the lining of our arteries. Damaged arterial linings initiate atherosclerosis. Known sources of this most harmful cholesterol include pancake and custard mixes, parmesan cheese, lard, and ice cream. Eating foods high in antioxidants (plant foods) helps neutralize these kinds of dangerous free radicals.

What are some practical ways to lower cholesterol?

Blood cholesterol levels are largely determined by what we eat. If you

CORONARY RISK AND CHOLESTEROL

500% Rise

Incidence per 1,000 population Coronary Death Rate/100

Cholesterol (mg%)

Lifestyle Medicine Institute

CHOLESTEROL

CHOLESTEROL CONTENT IN FOODS

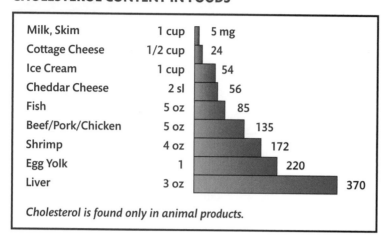

Milk, Skim	1 cup	5 mg
Cottage Cheese	1/2 cup	24
Ice Cream	1 cup	54
Cheddar Cheese	2 sl	56
Fish	5 oz	85
Beef/Pork/Chicken	5 oz	135
Shrimp	4 oz	172
Egg Yolk	1	220
Liver	3 oz	370

Cholesterol is found only in animal products.

are serious about lowering your cholesterol, follow these guidelines:

- **Eat less cholesterol.** Reduce the usual amount of 400 milligrams of cholesterol eaten to less than 50 milligrams a day, or better yet, to zero. Markedly reduce meat, especially organ meats and sausages, egg yolks and most dairy products; ideally, stop them altogether.
- **Eat much less fat.** Saturated fats and trans fats push the liver into overdrive in making cholesterol. These fats are more potent in raising blood cholesterol levels than the cholesterol we eat.
  - ~ Saturated fats are solid at room temperature (butter, lard) and are prominently found in animal products.
  - ~ Trans fats are formed when oils are partially hydrogenated to make them more "spreadable." They are found in margarines, many fast foods, and processed foods.
  - ~ Polyunsaturated (liquid) fats don't directly raise blood cholesterol levels, but they relate to certain adult cancers and overweight.
- **Eat less animal protein.** Homocysteine levels rise after a meal rich in animal protein, and these

elevated levels have been associated with increased cholesterol and an increased risk of coronary heart disease.

- **Eat more fiber.** Soluble fibers, plentifully found in oats, beans, and fruits, bind to cholesterol and bile acids in the intestines and prevent them from being reabsorbed into the bloodstream. Eating more of these fiber-rich foods can lower blood cholesterol levels as much as 10 percent.
- **Medications.** While the Optimal Diet will reduce high blood cholesterol by an average of 15 to 25 percent within four to eight weeks, cholesterol-lowering medications may be needed for a few who may not respond to the lifestyle measures. Be sure to check this with your physician.

Will these measures help raise HDL, the good cholesterol?

They will lower the LDL/HDL ratio, which will decrease cardiovascular risk.

You can raise HDL by losing excess weight, exercising daily, and eliminating smoking. Of course, if you bring down your LDL levels, then you won't have to worry so much about increasing your HDL, because the HDL derives its clinical significance largely from the amount of LDL. The higher the LDL, the more HDL is needed to be cardioprotective. The lower the LDL, the less HDL is needed.

Just remember, blood cholesterol levels are directly affected by the richness of the diet. A diet very low in fat (under 15 percent of calories) and high in fiber has been shown to lower most blood cholesterol levels by 15 to 25 percent in 30 days.

If you don't know what your blood cholesterol is, *run*, don't walk, to the nearest checkpoint. If the result is over 160 mg% (4.1 mmol/L), it's time to get serious!

NOTES

Application

Blood cholesterol levels are the most important factors in determining a person's risk for developing cardiovascular disease. A diet high in fat and animal products raises cholesterol levels. The opposite is also true. A diet very low in fat and cholesterol and high in fiber has been shown to lower high blood cholesterol levels on average 15 to 25 percent in 30 days.

Blood Cholesterol Level

All too often the first sign of heart disease is sudden death. The best way to assess the risk of heart disease before disaster strikes is by looking at the blood cholesterol profile. This profile is the single most important predictor of heart disease.

Do you know your blood cholesterol level? If you don't, make an appointment with your doctor to find out. The procedure is simple. But more important, what you learn could save your life.

What is your blood cholesterol level? _____
What is your blood LDL cholesterol? _____
What is your blood LDL/HDL ratio? _____

Take Aggressive Action

If you don't find yourself inside the safety zone with a blood cholesterol level below 160 mg% (4.1mmol/L), don't despair. It is time to take aggressive action. You can lower your cholesterol level by making important lifestyle changes.

Six Ways to Lower Cholesterol Levels

Here are six prescriptions that will help lower your cholesterol level. Put a checkmark by the ones you are already working on. Below each item, write ways you might achieve that objective. After you're done, review this chapter to see how your answers match.

> It used to be that no self-respecting food lover would be caught dead caring about fat grams and food groups. No more. Today's true gourmets are showing America how delicious healthy cooking can be.

Eat Less Cholesterol:

_____
_____
_____

Eat Less Fat:

_____
_____
_____

Lose Excess Weight:

_____
_____
_____

Eat More Fiber:

_____
_____

Exercise More:

_____
_____

Medications (if necessary):

_____
_____

Your Challenge

Review your list of things you can do to lower your blood cholesterol level and begin acting on these strategies.

Inedible, Indigestible, Essential

Juices are actually fruits and vegetables robbed of their fiber.

There is part of our food that goes right through our bodies and into the toilet without ever being used. What a downer! What a waste! Right?

Wrong! That was the thinking, even of many scientists, until the early 1970s. But now we know that fiber is like a general—it controls many body processes.

Just what is fiber?

Fiber is the framework of plants. Because it passes through the body without being absorbed by the blood, fiber was long thought to be of no value. Removing it from food, however, increased the caloric density of food and the efficiency and speed with which it was absorbed into the bloodstream. Removing fiber from the food also prolonged the food's shelf life.

The many kinds of fiber fall into two basic groups—those that dissolve in water (soluble fiber) and those that don't (insoluble fiber).

What does fiber do?

Fiber is involved in many of the body's digestive and metabolic processes. Here are some of them:

- **Insoluble fiber** absorbs and holds water—from four to six times its own volume—creating soft, spongy masses in the stomach and in the small and large intestines. The result? A sense of fullness occurs much sooner than with low-fiber foods, protecting against overeating and aiding in weight control.

  The fiber masses, acting like soaked-up sponges, fill the intestines more completely and stimulate them to lively activity. Instead of idling for several days in the gastrointestinal tract in

Focus on whole-grain cereals and breads, fresh fruit and vegetables, and plenty of beans and other legumes. This is the healthiest, safest, cheapest, and best way to get the fiber you need.

compacted clumps, as low-fiber foods do, the spongy masses pass along much more quickly and are evacuated within 24 to 36 hours.

This action cures most constipation and significantly relieves problems with hemorrhoids and diverticular disease.

- Because of the shorter transit time, less putrefaction (decomposition of organic material) in the intestines occurs and there is less time for carcinogens and other harmful end products of digestion to irritate the bowel walls. The fiber also provides insulation against damaging food residues. These fiber-related actions may explain the lower colon cancer rates among people with higher fiber intakes.
- Fiber also slows down the rate at which nutrients enter the bloodstream. This helps smooth out the ups and downs of blood sugar levels and provides more consistent energy throughout the day. A stabilized blood sugar relieves most hypoglycemia (low blood sugar) and aids in the control of diabetes (high blood sugar).
- **Soluble fiber,** on the other hand, is the type that affects

blood cholesterol levels. Soluble fiber attaches itself to cholesterol and other by-products of fat digestion, and pulls them right out of the body. Without soluble fiber's action, most of the leftover cholesterol would be reabsorbed into the blood-

Fiber isn't something you can sprinkle on a plate of steak and eggs and make it OK.

stream, adding to the already-high levels found in those following a Western diet. Soluble fiber is especially plentiful in fruit, beans, and oats.

Where else do you find this seeming miracle worker?

Fiber is abundant in all unrefined plant foods. Eating a variety of fruits, whole grains, vegetables, and legumes (beans, lentils, peas) assures a plentiful supply of the many varieties of fiber the body needs.

Most people are surprised to learn that animal foods do not contain any fiber. And since meat, poultry, fish,

eggs, and dairy products make up more than 40 percent of the calories of the typical Western diet, and much of the rest comes from sugars and other refined foods, the result is that those following a Western diet will get only about one third of the fiber they need each day.

What about juicers? That seems like a good way to get lots of fruits and vegetables.

The commercials have certainly been convincing. Piles of great-looking fresh produce are fed into a little machine, and presto— beautiful juice!

Across the country busy people, accustomed to technological wonder and dedicated to health improvement have been welcoming yet another exciting shortcut to the good life: fruit and vegetable juicers.

But do they live up to their claims?

Yes and no. Yes, they produce a nutritious drink; but no, most do not live up to the health claims that are all too often made for them.

While juice machines deliver a product that is fairly rich in nutrients, most do so at the expense of valuable food fiber. Ten pounds of fresh

The Anti-Breast Cancer Diet

Breast cancer is a hormonally driven tumor, and estrogen is the fuel it needs to grow. When too much estrogen reaches body receptors, the risk rises for these tumors to grow.

The anti-breast cancer diet includes 30 to 50 grams of fiber, which interrupts many of the steps of estrogen activity.

FIBER

FIBER IN FOODS

Food	Portion	Fiber (gm)
Cereal, high in bran	1 cup	20
Garbanzo beans	1 cup	16
Apple	large	9
Broccoli, cooked	1 stalk	9
Beans and peas, cooked	1 cup	8
Whole-wheat bread	3 slices	8
Grains and cereals	1 cup	5
Berries	1/2 cup	5
Steak	5 oz.	0
Chicken	5 oz.	0
Fish	5 oz.	0
Cheese	1 oz.	0

"Beware of meats and cheeses.
They are totally devoid of fiber."

It would take a whole bottle
of fiber pills to supply the fiber
contained in a bowl of whole-grain
cereal topped with strawberries.

produce may yield two quarts of delicious juice. But with most juices, nearly all the precious fiber, which the body so badly needs, is in the five or six pounds of pulp that usually go out with the garbage.

The process is reminiscent of the flour mills of 100 years ago that began removing bran and germ (fiber and nutrients) from grains, leaving low-fiber, nutrient-poor residues, such as white flour and white rice. Unfortunately these foods are still the mainstay of much of the current world population.

For people who find it hard to chew fresh food, certain juice machines that retain food fiber are available. The product is thick, like pudding, but can be diluted like ordinary juice concentrate.

Wouldn't it be a good idea to add wheat, oat, rice, and other brans to our food?

Remember the oat bran craze a few years back?

Oat bran was billed as a quick fix for pulling down stubborn cholesterol levels. Foodmakers jumped to take advantage of the windfall. An oatmeal war broke out. Oat bran became scarce, and the price shot up. Then some new studies appeared, which cast doubt on these claims. Besides, people were getting tired of mush and muffins. The new studies didn't debunk oat bran as a valuable cholesterol-lowering food. What the studies did show was that a big bowl of any hot starchy cereal, eaten for breakfast, would displace an appreciable amount of bacon, eggs, sausage, croissants, and other foods that kick in the liver's cholesterol-producing machinery. And oat bran fiber held no advantage over soluble fibers in other foods, such as beans and fruit.

These observations make sense. Any dietary change in which low-fat, starchy, no-cholesterol plant foods replace high-fat, high-cholesterol animal foods has been repeatedly shown to be effective in lowering cholesterol levels.

You're confusing me. Are you saying we shouldn't eat these brans?

Not really. It's just that people need to realize that extracted brans are not magical potions that they can gulp down and expect to ream out their blood vessels and intestines. People who eat lots of plant foods will get the fiber they need, both soluble and insoluble.

Adding wheat bran can be helpful to sedentary people on limited diets. But most people don't need fiber pills, extracted brans, and other expensive supplements.

It would take a whole bottle of fiber pills to supply the fiber contained in a bowl of whole-grain cereal topped with strawberries. Fiber is not something you can sprinkle on a plate of steak and eggs and make it OK.

Fiber-poor foods are hazardous to your health. Don't be misled by gimmicks that tamper with the balance of natural foods.

Focus on whole-grain cereals and breads, fresh fruit and vegetables, and plenty of beans and other legumes. This is the healthiest, safest, cheapest, and best way to get the fiber you need.

Application

Fiber plays a crucial role in weight control, diabetes, and digestion. It also helps protect against colon cancer. Eating a variety of unrefined foods is the best way to provide your body with the fiber it needs.

Addition and Subtraction

What did you have for supper last night? List everything you ate:

_____

_____

_____

_____

Now, put a plus sign in front of everything that contained whole grains, vegetables, legumes, or fruit. When you have finished, put a minus sign in front of everything that contained sugar, meat, white flour, milk, butter, oil, fat, eggs, or processed foods. It's OK if you end up with several pluses and minuses in front of a single item.

What It All Means

The principle is simple. For every plus, the food you ate added fiber to your diet. For every minus, a refined food or an animal product added little, if any. Too many minus signs on your list? Then it's time to make some adjustments to your menu.

The Western Diet

When it comes to dietary fiber the Western diet is full of minuses. First, its focus on meat and other animal products provides a shaky foundation. Any food that comes from an animal has absolutely no fiber. Zero.

Second, about half of the calories in the standard American diet are empty calories. An empty calorie provides no vitamins, minerals, or fiber.

Your Challenge

Start replacing fiber-free foods with fiber-filled foods in your diet. Begin with this flavorful dish:

Black Beans Over Rice

Beans

1¼ c black beans	5 c water
1 clove garlic, minced	1/2 tsp salt
1 c onion, chopped	1 green pepper, chopped
1 onion, peeled and stuck with 3 whole cloves	

Cook beans in Crockpot until they start to get tender. Add garlic and clove-studded onion and salt. Cook 1 hour more.

Sauté onions and green peppers in water or broth. Take the whole onion with cloves from beans and discard. Stir in sautéed onions and green peppers.

Rice

4 c cooked brown rice (1½ c uncooked rice)

Salsa

16-oz can of unsalted, unpeeled tomatoes, drained

3/4 c diced red onion	2 cloves garlic, minced
1 Tbsp lemon juice	1/2 c parsley, chopped fine

In small bowl, break up tomatoes with spoon. Add other salsa ingredients, cover, and refrigerate to let flavors blend. Serve beans over cooked rice. Top with salsa.

THE STANDARD AMERICAN DIET

Empty Calories as a Percent of Total Calories	
Refined sugar	21%
Visible fats and oils	20%
Alcohol (men)	9%
Total Empty Calories	**50%**

Overfed and undernourished!

The Salt Assault

We can't live without it—but too much brings a host of troubles.

N orth Americans eat 10 times more salt than they need. And they pay for it with high blood pressure, heart failure, and other problems related to fluid retention.

Don't we need salt?

Salt contains two minerals, sodium and chloride. Sodium is the important one; every cell contains sodium, as do all body fluids. We couldn't live without it. But while it is essential for body functions, sodium can also cause trouble.

How does salt raise blood pressure?

Excess sodium can stay in body tissues and hold extra water. This causes edema and swelling. This, in turn, applies pressure to the large network of capillaries, which then forces blood pressure to increase in order to get the blood pushed through the resistant circulatory channels. The higher blood pressure, in turn, increases stress on the heart. Every third American adult now has an elevated blood pressure. In those over age 65 the figures rise to 70 percent.

The average salt intake in Japan is even higher than in North America—and so is the prevalence of hypertension. Stroke, a complication of hypertension, is the leading cause of death in Japan.

In other societies, such as those in rural Uganda or the Amazon basin, where salt intake is very low, hypertension is virtually unknown even in advanced age. Dr. Lot Page, a respected researcher, stated categorically, "Without exception, low-blood-pressure societies are low-salt societies. Conversely, mass hypertension follows mass salt consumption."

Is this true for everyone?

Not everyone is salt-sensitive. Some people can eat all they want without ill effects. Most Americans, however, have some vulnerability to salt, and there is no satisfactory test for identifying them.

Salt-sensitive people retain sodium, which causes fluid retention to dilute the sodium. Many people carry five to seven extra pounds of water weight because of excess salt in their bodies. Decreasing salt intake allows the body to shed the excess water.

Some 30 million Americans with mild essential hypertension could normalize their blood pressures by cutting their salt intake to less than 5,000 milligrams (1 teaspoon) a day.

Besides weight and blood pressure control, such a low-salt diet favorably affects the premenstrual syndrome (PMS), certain headaches, and some depressions. And it reduces the waterlogging in chronic heart failure.

What about water pills?

Water pills successfully lower blood pressure by eliminating salt and extra water. But research has shown that some of these medications may possibly contribute to heart disease by increasing cholesterol levels 5 to 10 percent. Over time these drugs may also damage the kidneys, promote gout, and accelerate diabetes. Eliminating extra water by natural means would be the safer way to go. And it would cost less!

Don't people who take diuretics for high blood pressure have to take them for life?

That was yesterday's news. The word today is that up to 80 percent of mild and moderate hypertensives could be eased off their blood pressure pills in response to a very low-salt, low-fat diet combined with weight loss and daily walking.

But I can't stand saltless food!

Salt preferences are not inborn. Saltiness is a learned habit, and eating salty foods fuels the craving. Salt masks natural flavors. Shake the habit by seasoning with herbs and spices. Give yourself three weeks.

After that, even so-called normal foods will begin to taste salty. For the diehards, use salt substitutes.

What are some high-sodium foods to avoid?

Watch out for baking soda, baking powder, MSG (monosodium glutamate), salty snacks, and anything

Healthy by choice, not by chance!

pickled. Eat less processed foods, baked goods, meats, dairy products, and certain presweetened cereals. Especially shun canned vegetables unless labeled "no salt added." One tablespoon of canned peas contains as much sodium as five pounds of fresh peas!

How much salt is safe to eat?

Most people are genuinely amazed at how little salt the body actually needs in a day—an average of about one gram or 1,000 mg,

which is one fifth of a teaspoon of salt.

However, if this is too drastic a change for you, then concentrate on cutting back. Instead of two teaspoons (10 grams), limit yourself to one teaspoon (five grams) of salt a day. This is a reasonably safe limit for most people.

Here are some ideas to help you decrease the salt in your diet:
- Eat lots of fresh, raw foods, both fruits and vegetables. They need no added salt. They also increase potassium stores, which help lower blood pressure.
- If you need them, look for unsalted snacks.
- Undercook vegetables and eat them a bit crispy. They will require less salt.
- Toast (dextrinize) bread and cereals for added flavor.
- Learn to flavor foods with lemon juice, fresh herbs, parsley, tarragon, garlic, and onions, instead of with salt.
- Take advantage of the excellent

FOOD PROCESSING—HIDDEN SALT

Food Natural State	Salt (mg)	Food Commercial, Processed	Salt (mg)
Apple (1 fresh)	5	Apple Pie (1 slice)	500
White Beans (1 cup)	12	Chili and Beans (1 cup)	3,000
Rice, brown (1 cup)	12	Rice-A-Roni Pilaf (1 cup)	120
Wheat Flakes (2 oz)	20	Wheaties (2 oz)	1,050
Potato (1 fresh, 5 oz)	20	Potato Chips (5 oz)	2,750
Tomato (1 fresh)	35	Tomato Sauce (1/2 cup)	1,500
Beef, lean (3 oz)	140	Corned Beef (3 oz)	1,685
Milk (1 cup)	300	Cheese, Amer. (2 slices)	1,800
Chicken (8 oz)	300	Kentucky Fried Chicken (three-piece dinner)	5,600

SALT "BOMBS"

Condiment	Amount	Salt (mg)
Ketchup	2 tsp	950
Italian Dressing	3 tsp	1,350
Soy Sauce	1 tsp	2,300
Dill Pickle	1 large	2,600
Garlic Salt	1 tsp	4,500
Salt	1 tsp	5,000

Remember: Most of our salt comes from processed food, from crinkly bags, fast foods, and restaurant foods. The saltshaker actually plays only a minor role.

The taste for salt is not inborn. Saltiness is something we've learned, and eating salty foods fuels the craving.

The sodium in salt (Sodium Chloride) is responsible for the effect on blood pressure. Every gram of salt contains .4 gm of sodium. Or every 1,000 mg of salt contains 400 mg of Sodium. To convert salt to sodium, multiply salt times .4. To convert sodium to salt, divide sodium by .4.

salt-free gourmet cookbooks available on the market today.

Those nutrition labels are not easy to understand. Any Suggestions?

When it comes to the salt content, you will find the sodium content to be listed. It is listed per servings of food. A simple and magical rule is this: try to keep the number of milligrams of sodium in the neighborhood of the numbers of calories per serving. If the calories per serving is 300, try to keep the sodium content between 250 and 350 mg – and you'll come out ok. For instance, if you eat 2,000 calories for the whole day, you'll have ingested about 2,000 mg of sodium which is 5,000 mg of salt, or 5 gm. You accomplished your sodium goal for that day!

The average American consumes 8 pounds of salt a year. Reducing this to three pounds would be a major step toward better health.

NOTES

We eat 10 times more salt than is needed. High blood pressure, heart failure, and stroke are among the sad results. By avoiding highly salted foods and re-educating ourselves to enjoy meals with little or no added salt, we take a giant step toward better health.

What Do You Have to Lose?

You can shed excess water, lower your blood pressure, protect yourself against stroke and heart disease—all this just by reducing the salt in your diet. It's a smart move. Are you ready to give it a try?

Cooking the Salt-free Way

It takes about three weeks for your tastes to adjust to a low-salt diet. During that time food can taste pretty bland. Stick with it, however, and you will be rewarded when the delicious, natural flavors of food come out of hiding.

Herbs Instead of Salt

Seasoning with herbs is an important skill for the health-conscious cook to master. Here are some suggestions to spice up your meals:

1. Use no more than one-fourth teaspoon of dried herbs, or three-fourths teaspoon of fresh herbs, for a dish that serves four people.
2. To soups and stews that are cooked a long time, add herbs during the last 15 minutes of cooking.
3. When cooking vegetables or making sauces and gravies, cook herbs along with them.
4. To cold foods, such as tomato juice, salad dressings, and cottage cheese, add herbs several hours before serving. Storing these foods in the refrigerator for three to four hours deepens the flavor.
5. Remember that the correct combination of herbs and spices is the one that tastes best to you.
6. A very versatile seasoning is *Mrs. Dash*. Use the one without salt and low in pepper.
7. Don't overseason. Vegetables have wonderful flavors in their own right.

Seasoning Vegetables

Vegetables play a central role in the Optimal Diet. Here is a list of vegetables with some seasoning suggestions:

Suggested Seasonings for Vegetables

Asparagus: lemon juice, chives, thyme, tarragon.
Beans, dried: bay leaf, garlic, marjoram, onion, oregano.
Beans, green: basil, dill seed, thyme, onion, tarragon.
Beets: lemon juice or lemon peel.
Broccoli: lemon juice, dill, oregano.
Cabbage: creole cabbage with tomatoes, green pepper, garlic, and onion.
Carrots: parsley, mint, dill weed, lemon peel, sesame seed.
Cauliflower: Italian seasonings, paprika, sesame seed.
Celery: stir-fry with low-salt soy sauce, sesame seeds, and tomato.
Corn: bell pepper, pimiento, tomatoes, chives.
Okra: try broiling for a crisp texture.
Peas: fresh mushrooms, pearl onions, water chestnuts.
Potatoes: parsley, chopped green pepper, onion, chives.
Spinach: lemon juice, rosemary.
Squash: bake with chopped apple and lemon juice.
Tomatoes: basil; sprinkle with curry powder; broil with mushrooms, green pepper, and onion.

Your Challenge

Use herbs instead of salt when you cook. Experiment with new seasonings for vegetables. The switch will increase the flavor of your food and decrease your risk of high blood pressure and stroke.

Megadosing on Micronutrients

Never before has something we need so little of been sold so big—$25 billion big!

Thousands of people, attempting to become healthier, may be filling their bodies with large doses of vitamin and mineral supplements that can be dangerous.

I've never seen anything on the subject. How is one supposed to know?

That's the problem. For years we have been given minimum requirements and Recommended Daily Intakes (RDI) for most vitamins and a few of the minerals, but no safe upper limits of dosages have been established. This is because, so far, vitamins and minerals are classified under foods rather than drugs, and thus are not subjected to the extensive scrutiny and testing that drugs receive.

What kinds of damage can result from excessive intake of vitamins and minerals?

One danger is the notion that large doses may prevent serious diseases, such as cancer, heart disease, and osteoporosis. Actually, large supplemental doses of single nutrients may interfere with the absorption of other nutrients. For example, high levels of iron appear to reduce zinc absorption, while high intakes of zinc may impair copper absorption.

Several vitamins are soluble only in fat. Overloads cannot be excreted, but are picked up and stored in the liver. Toxic doses of vitamin A (20 times the RDI dose) can produce throbbing headaches, dry skin (with cracked lips), joint pain, and loss of hair. Pregnant women who take megadoses of vitamin A may endanger their babies.

Other fat-soluble vitamins are vitamins D, E, and K.

Then we have the water-soluble vitamins (B complex and C). They were long thought to do no harm because the body could eliminate the excesses through the urine. But that rule went out the window a few years back when megadoses of vitamin B$_6$ were shown to produce disturbances in the nervous system. Obviously excessive doses of the water-soluble vitamins have been shown to cause the body to become very wasteful of these nutrients. And

More on Vitamins

Large studies have revealed some controversial findings. Sometimes the vitamin supplement works, and at other times it doesn't. It appears that many vitamins in their natural food context are actually biologically activated, boosted by bio-cofactors that surround them. Once these special "boosters" are removed by extracting the vitamin, or making them in the laboratory, their potency can be affected in a major way.

megadoses of vitamin C may cause kidney stones.

Another worry is that the long-term effects of megadoses are unknown. We are taking chances. Indiscriminate use can amount to over-the-counter drug abuse.

What's the safest way to get vitamins and minerals?

Ideally, we should get our micronutrients from our food. Natural foods are heavily laden with vitamins and minerals in amounts and forms that allow the body to pick and choose what it needs. Once we separate nutrients from food, once we concentrate anything in the food chain, we run the risk of upsetting this natural balance.

What about people on limited food intakes, and others who pay little attention to their nutrition?

Scientists are not too concerned about people taking a daily multi-vitamin tablet that supplies the recommended daily intake for several vitamins and minerals. Supplements at reasonable levels may provide assurances in marginal situations.

Strict vegans (no animal products at all) may need to supplement their diets with vitamin B_{12}. This vitamin is present in soy sauces. It is also added

Vitamin D: 15 minutes of sunlight to the face or arms each day will give you all that you need.

to certain commercial food products like cereals and soy milk. Just to be sure, some vegans take a B_{12} tablet (50 micrograms) once a week. (This tablet must be dissolved under the tongue to be absorbed into the bloodstream.)

But don't extra vitamins help with stress and increase energy levels?

It is difficult to find consistent documented evidence that vitamin and mineral supplements make people more energetic or give them an edge over handling their stress. These micronutrients do not function in a magical manner. In excess, they will not push the pace of the body's biological reactions any more than extra gas in the tank will make a car go faster than its engine capacity allows. Energy comes from fuel foods (carbohydrates such as grains, legumes, potatoes). It doesn't come from vitamins and minerals.

While we need these micronutrients to live healthily we need them in very minuscule amounts. People don't realize that they can put all the vitamins they need for a whole month into a thimble—easily.

What about herbs? Do they live up to the hype?

A pinch of herbs, deftly chosen, can perk up a meal. Try flavoring your foods with herbs, and you'll be able to cut down on salt, even omit it altogether.

Why is there so much controversy about herbs?

Controversies develop when

herbs are used as medicines. People today, looking for safer treatments, often turn to herbs. While most of the commonly used herbs appear to be quite safe, there are some cautions people need to be aware of.

The biggest problem is that herbs have not undergone the rigorous testing required of other pharmaceuticals. Like vitamins, they are classed as foods, and the FDA is not allowed to test them.

This means that for most herbs, the safe upper limit of dosage has not been determined, nor have their side effects, toxicity, long-term safety, and efficacy been scientifically studied. It also means that no one is checking to see exactly what compounds the herb contains, if it contains as much as it claims, or anything at all.

Herbs with enough pharmacological activity to be useful are often the ones that pose the greatest hazards. Biologic activity is a two-edged sword. Here are several ways the use of herbs may become hazardous:

- The quantity of active herb in a preparation is often extremely variable for the following reasons:
  - ~ Improper preparation
  - ~ Plant variation
  - ~ Choice of the plant part used
  - ~ Fraud
  - ~ Soil conditions
- The herb preparation may not contain the needed ingredient for the illness being treated.
- The herb preparation may interact in a harmful way with prescription drugs or may be harmful itself.
- The preparation may have more than one active ingredient, as well as other compounds that vary in chemical composition from batch to batch.

That seems like a lot of bad news!

Just remember: be careful. It is a mistake to assume that because something is natural, it is also safe.

On the other hand, toxic reactions to herbs are relatively rare, while serious reactions and complications to conventional medicines are all too common.

Perhaps someday the Federal Drug Administration will create a new Division of Natural Therapeutics. Then we could feel a bit more secure about our supplements.

How Do We Decide?

With so many people slanting the health news for their own purposes, how do we know what to believe? Good common sense is one answer. When you read about the results of a study or hear the claims of an advertiser, ask yourself the following questions:

Believability Checklist

1. Who is making this claim? Be suspicious if it is the producer of the product.

2. What do they have to gain publicizing this information? What is their motive?

3. Do other studies agree with these claims, or is this an exception or "new" finding being picked up by the media? News media love a sensational story. As a result, they often publish the results of flawed or biased studies.

4. Does the claim sound like magic? If it sounds too good to be true, chances are it is.

5. Is a drug or food touted as reversing a chronic condition brought on by long-term lifestyle patterns? Beware of the quick fix.

6. Does the claim contradict the principles of balance and common sense?

Preoccupation with new discoveries and "quick fixes" focuses attention away from the need for a healthy lifestyle and well-balanced diet. The best place to get your vitamins and minerals is from fresh, whole foods. They're packed with the things your body needs for good health. Megadoses of supplements can be toxic. Don't upset your body's natural balance by taking too much of a good thing.

Health Doesn't Come in a Bottle

No potion or pill can undo a lifetime of neglected health. Despite the claims of advertisers eager to make their fortune selling high-priced supplements, vitamin and mineral megadoses are not miracle cures.

Does This Make Sense?

People in industrialized countries spend billions on processed and packaged foods that have many of their nutrients removed, and then turn around and pay fantastic prices for food supplements. Wouldn't it make more sense to eat the original, nutrient-packed foods instead?

You can't eat whole foods without getting a sizable dose of vitamins and minerals. For example, a medium-sized potato contains 40 percent of the recommended daily intake of vitamin C, plus fiber, niacin, and potassium. It's a natural multivitamin.

Relax and Enjoy

All fresh fruits, whole grains, and vegetables provide an abundance of nutrients. If you eat a variety of these foods every day, your need for vitamins, minerals, and fiber is easily met.

Your Challenge

Put a permanent checkmark next to broccoli on your shopping list. One cup of this leafy green vegetable, cooked, has 165 percent of the RDI for vitamin C, 50 percent for vitamin A, 20 percent for calcium, plus iron, B vitamins, potassium, and other minerals.

SOME SOURCES OF SELECTED NUTRIENTS

Nutrient	Sources
Vitamin A	Dark-green, yellow, and orange vegetables and fruit.
Vitamin B$_1$	Whole-grain products, peas, beans, wheat germ, potatoes, and leafy vegetables.
Vitamin B$_2$	Green leafy vegetables, whole-grain products, and prunes.
Vitamin B$_3$	Whole-grain and enriched breads and cereals, legumes, potatoes, and green vegetables.
Vitamin B$_{12}$	Dairy products (nonfat), soy sauce, enriched commercial products, certain cereals, milk substitutes, etc.
Vitamin C	Cantaloupe, lemons, grapefruit, oranges, strawberries, raw cabbage, sweet peppers, tomatoes, and potatoes.
Vitamin D	Direct sunshine and fortified milks.
Vitamin E	Whole grains, leafy vegetables, dairy products, and sunflower seeds.
Iron	Legumes, whole-grain cereals and breads, dried fruits, and green leafy vegetables.
Calcium	Mustard, kale, turnip tops, cabbage, broccoli, whole-grain products, citrus fruits, tofu, skim milk, and milk substitutes.

With their penchant for taking vitamin C, Americans probably have the most expensive urine in the world. As a rule of thumb: Once the tissues have been saturated with a water-soluble vitamin, the body flushes out any excess.

NOTES

Nature's Cancer Fighters

Nutritionists and mothers have been telling us for years that vitamin pills and supplements are no substitute for eating our vegetables. Now scientists are finding out why. It turns out that fruits and vegetables are loaded with compounds called phytochemicals and antioxidants that demonstrably lower the risk of cancer.

These phytochemicals—are they related to vitamins?

No, they are not vitamins or minerals. They aren't even nutrients in the strict sense of the word. Phyto is Latin for plant. These are natural chemicals found only in plants. These food chemicals cannot be obtained from animal products.

What makes these substances so exciting is that study after study continues to reveal the many cancer-protective benefits of the different phytochemicals.

How many of these chemicals have been discovered so far?

When you hear reports about every carrot and every tomato containing hundreds of these compounds, you'll get some idea of the complexity of these findings. They are opening up a whole new dimension in our understanding of nutrition.

How much can a person expect to reduce the risk of cancer by eating more fruits and vegetables?

Actually quite a bit. More than 400 major scientific studies over the past 25 years have consistently shown that high plant food eaters are about half as likely to have cancer as those who eat few plant foods. This is also true for heart disease, adult diabetes, and certain other lifestyle diseases. Eating a variety of vegetables and fruits daily

> God said to Adam: "You will eat the plants of the field."
> —Genesis 3:18

ensures an adequate intake of most micronutrients, dietary fibers, and a host of essential nonnutrient substances. Increased fruit and vegetable consumption can help displace foods usually high in saturated and trans fats, sugar, and cholesterol.

Do we know how phytochemicals protect against cancer?

Researchers suggest that phytochemicals usually work either as blocking agents or suppressing agents.

- Blocking agents work on the carcinogens (cancer-causing compounds). They prevent them from affecting the body's cells. For example:
  - ~ Indoles found in cruciferous vegetables (cabbage, cauliflower, broccoli) work as blocking agents by increasing colon enzymes that can deactivate some of these carcinogens.
  - ~ Others block the ability of bacteria to attach themselves to the surface of the cell.
- Suppressing agents work on the body's own cells, combating malignant changes that have been started by free radicals or carcinogens.
  - ~ They can slow tumor growth by suppressing the cancer cells' ability to reproduce.
  - ~ They can suppress certain enzymes that cancer cells need in order to grow.

Do some fruits and vegetables contain more potent cancer-fighters than others?

Some of them do seem to stand out, although this probably reflects the fact that these foods have been studied more extensively than others.

- For colon cancers, it's the cruciferous vegetables.
- A high fruit and carrot intake appears to decrease the risk of lung cancers significantly.
- Research subjects eating one or more onions a day were found to have only half the stomach cancer risk of those who never ate onions.
- Soy, a more recent star on the food scene, is a veritable gold mine of cancer-protective phytochemicals. Studies suggest that soy foods decrease cancer risk at many sites, including breast, colon, rectum, lung, and stomach.

Despite such findings, most scientists feel that the lower cancer risk is really associated with eating a wide variety of fruits and vegetables rather than isolating certain ones.

How many fruits and vegetables should we be eating to make a substantial difference?

The American Institute for Cancer Research recommends a minimum of nine servings a day.

This is pretty radical considering how few fruits and vegetables most people in North America actually eat. Some don't eat any at all!

Some good news about phytochemicals is that you don't have to eat the foods raw to get the benefits. While a few of these compounds lose a fraction of their effect when cooked, most are heat-stable. In some instances cooking actually frees up some of the compounds, making them more effective. Also, it doesn't seem to matter whether the vegetables are canned, frozen, juiced, or peeled. Most survive boiling, microwaving, baking, pickling, and drying.

What about antioxidants? How do they differ from phytochemicals?

Like phytochemicals, antioxidants are also natural chemicals found in food, but they are not limited to

Do Americans Eat Their Disease-Prevention Foods?

- **80 percent** do not eat fruits or vegetables rich in carotenoids.
- **82 percent** do not eat cruciferous vegetables.
- **41 percent** do not eat any fruits.
- **72 percent** do not eat fruits or vegetables rich in vitamin C.
- **84 percent** do not eat high-fiber grain food, such as bread or cereal.

plant foods. The term *antioxidant* refers to a specific function they perform—they help the body dispose of free radicals that can genetically damage normal cells and set the stage for cancer and increased aging.

All matter is made up of molecules, including every cell in our bodies. Normally every molecule has electrons in orbit around its nucleus. These electrons normally come in pairs. This makes the molecule stable.

Some molecules, however, have electrons that are not in pairs, leaving them extremely unstable. These molecules are called free radicals, and they have a powerful drive to acquire a partner. A free radical will grab an electron from a neighboring compound, causing it to become "oxidized." This newly "oxidized" compound has now become a free radical itself, which, in turn, looks for another electron to steal. The result is a chain reaction where oxidation and damage can spread from one molecule to the next until something stops the process. Substances that can stop this chain reaction are called antioxidants.

Can we do something to prevent our bodies from forming free radicals?

Free radicals are not all bad. For example, one of the ways the body destroys poisons is through a system that uses oxidation reactions and free radicals. Free radicals are also essential for effective destruction of germs by the body's white blood cells.

However, free radicals can be extremely dangerous when present outside these functions. They have been found to have a role in at least 50 diseases. They have been observed to damage DNA and are linked to cancer. Because all living creatures produce free radicals—we cannot avoid them—it is important to strengthen our body's antioxidant defenses.

We hear so much about the vitamins A, C, and E as antioxidants. Are there others?

There are many more. The natural body hormone melatonin, for example, is a very active antioxidant. Many of the phytochemicals are also antioxidants. Some caution, however, should be kept in mind when dealing with antioxidants.

- Too large a dose of one antioxidant can suppress the action of another. For example, high doses of beta-carotene pills can deplete the body's supply of needed vitamin E.
- When taken alone, in high dosages, some antioxidants can become free radicals.
- Preformed vitamin A is toxic in large doses, whereas beta-carotene and its relatives, the carotenoids, can be converted to vitamin A whenever the body needs it.
- Supplements do not furnish the same protection as does eating the foods. For example, beta-carotene tablets do not contain the many other carotenoids the body uses. The vitamin E commonly found in supplements is the wrong kind for some body needs.
- Research on antioxidants is done with foods, not supplements.
- The Federal Drug Administration is not allowed to test supplements, because they are considered foods. So we do not know for sure the toxic range, side effects, or efficacy, or even that the supplement contains what it is advertised to contain.

Are you saying we shouldn't use supplements?

No, just that we must be very careful about how we use them. If used, they should be taken in modest doses. More of a good thing is not always better. Besides, with so many different compounds having so many different actions, increasing the intake of certain ones over others can upset the balance of the system, and possibly suppress the effectiveness of compounds not yet discovered.

Perhaps someday Americans will realize that swallowing pills instead of eating the food is sheer nutritional madness—and slow suicide. But as long as hope persists that a special pill, a magic bullet, will appear someday to take care of everything, we will continue to be bombarded by every new "discovery" that comes along.

This is a relatively new field with seemingly endless challenges. We will continue to learn about these wondrous substances for years to come.

Application

Unrefined plant foods are found to contain substances that protect the body from cancer and other diseases. The best way to take advantage of this protection is to eat a wide variety of fruits, vegetables, and grains.

Plant sources of nutrition are generally modest in protein and reasonable in fat content; furthermore, they never contain any cholesterol. With our growing understanding of protein physiology, a plant-based diet has emerged as the optimum way to eat for those interested in longevity and the quality of living.

Following are lists of fruits and vegetables known to be especially high in phytochemicals and antioxidants. Check those that you eat fairly regularly.

Fruit
___ Cantaloupe
___ Strawberry
___ Plum
___ Orange
___ Red grapes
___ Kiwi
___ Pink grapefruit
___ White grapes
___ Bananas
___ Apple
___ Tomato

Vegetables
___ Soybeans
___ Garlic
___ Kale
___ Spinach
___ Brussel sprouts
___ Alfalfa sprouts
___ Broccoli
___ Beets
___ Red bell pepper
___ Onion
___ Corn

List below some new plant foods you would like to try this week:

_____
_____
_____
_____

A Good Rule of Thumb

Eat at least three different colors of fruits and vegetables every day.

THE OPTIMAL DIET

Legumes, Seeds, and Nuts | Fruits
Vegetables | Whole Grains

NOTES
_____
_____
_____
_____
_____
_____
_____
_____
_____
_____
_____
_____
_____
_____

In one year a typical American diet yields 270,000 fat calories. A starch-based diet will cut that figure to 73,000. As a result, you can eat more and not gain weight! Even five to 10 pounds of extra weight is associated with higher mortality rates. Almost any degree of overweight has an adverse effect on health and longevity.

AS BEFITS a country with 150,000 fast-food restaurants and 4 million food-vending machines, America is stomach and hips ahead of the rest of the world.

Weight Control

- Ads and Fads
- Diets
- Soft Drinks
- Snacks
- Fat Burner
- Calories
- Children
- Ideal Weight
- Breakfast
- Fail-safe Formula

When Success Is an Illusion

Losing weight can prove lifesaving, especially for people with diabetes, high blood pressure, and coronary heart disease.

The appeal is irresistible. "LOSE 10 POUNDS IN 10 DAYS—with a new, scientifically proven formula!" The struggling, discouraged, and overweight grasp at another straw. They need to believe.

Weight loss is weight loss, isn't it? Does it matter how a person loses it?

Most people who lose weight believe they are losing fat; in reality they may be losing mostly water plus muscle and other vital tissues.

People long for a safe diet pill, but so far this route has been anything but safe. Results are inconsistent and mostly disappointing. Some diet pills have caused permanent health damage, and a few have proved to be deadly.

Many diet plans include a diuretic (water pill). Since the body is about 70 percent water, it is relatively easy for such pills to remove several pounds of water quickly. The scales look good—for a few days. But gradually the body balances itself by replacing the water, and there goes the weight loss.

An overdose of protein will accomplish basically the same thing. The liver changes excess protein into blood urea nitrogen (BUN), which causes the kidneys to force water from the body. It takes much more water to wash out the products of excess protein metabolism than it does to take care of the breakdown products of either carbohydrates or fats.

Some quick-weight-loss diets take advantage of the fact that a high-protein intake can cause spectacular weight loss in a short time. This is a dangerous practice, however. That's why such diets are usually physician-supervised and limited to short periods of time, normally about two weeks. The scales show gratifyingly low numbers, but most of the weight returns in a short time as the body replaces lost water.

What other possible problems can such diets cause?

Many of the quickie diets drop daily intake of 1,800 to 2,500 calories to less than 500 calories a day. Some of these starvation diets may go as low as 300 to 400 calories. The body misreads this dramatic calorie drop as acute starvation and actually begins to digest its own protein (usually in the form of muscle) in an effort to protect more vital tissues. Careful testing has shown that weight loss on these diets can come from both fat and muscle tissues.

So beware! When you think you are losing 14 pounds of fat, for example, you could actually be losing five pounds of fat, one pound of protein tissue (muscle) and eight pounds of water.

If you feel you need to go on a diet, make sure that you get enough calories from protein and carbohydrates to prevent muscle tissue loss. For an average person this means at least 200 calories of protein (50 grams) and at least 600 calories of carbohydrate a day.

Can I really lose weight on such a gradual diet?

Moderately overweight people usually lose one to two pounds a week on a well-balanced diet; seriously overweight persons may lose a

> When you lose weight, you gain: energy, sex drive, happiness . . . life

little more. Slow, steady weight loss has many advantages over the radical diets: it does not throw the body into the mode of starvation metabolism; binges and failures are much less frequent; hunger becomes more manageable; and chances are good that the weight lost is really fat.

But perhaps the most important aspect of slower weight loss is that it allows time to establish new and more healthful habits of eating. A person must develop a better, healthier lifestyle for weight loss to have any chance of being permanent.

I'm desperate to lose weight; I have no patience with slow programs. Wouldn't quick weight loss be better than none at all?

Losing and regaining weight over and over is one of the most harmful things you can do to your body. The truth is that remaining overweight would be less harmful to overall health than this yo-yo effect. Repeated weight loss through crash diets, followed by regaining the weight, gradually depletes muscle tissue and adds fat tissue. And because muscle tissue is where fat is burned, you will become increasingly unable to lose weight.

Of even more concern are the psychological consequences. Enduring years of repeated failure and humiliation produces emotional scars that often remain for a lifetime. People seduced by the magic of quick weight loss do shed pounds initially; but they almost invariably end up weighing more than they did before.

This is not to minimize the fact that overweight persons carry in-

The Skinny on Cellulite

- Thigh creams haven't produced lasting results.
- There are no miracle pills. They only slim down your pocketbook.
- Liposuction is expensive. The fat goes, but not the dimpled skin.
- Massages, wraps and such—save your money!
- With a low-fat, reduced-calorie diet you'll lose one to two pounds a week, and reshape your cellulite.
- Best bet: low-fat *Optimal Diet* plus regular active exercise.

Diet Failure

Thirty years of a nationwide struggle against obesity have failed. In spite of a plethora of weight-loss programs, more than 90 percent regain the weight they lost within a year.

Looking at statistics and waist-lines—we are the butt of jokes around the world. Some reasons:

- Portion sizes border on the obscene—
  - ~ doughnuts the size of pie plates
  - ~ monster muffins
  - ~ 64-ounce soft drinks
  - ~ one-pound burritos
  - ~ McDonald's "original" 3.7-ounce burger is now the 5.3-ounce Angus Deluxe Burger.
- Americans are sedentary: 4.4 hours of daily TV, plus Internet use.
- Our food isn't served— it's shoveled!

creased health risks. They have more heart disease, hypertension, diabetes, gallbladder disease, and cancer than do people of normal weight. They also die sooner.

Don't become a slave to the scale, checking it daily for immediate results to problems that took years to develop. Get started on a healthful program. And be patient. It's the long haul that matters. The illusions will fade, but the eventual rewards will be solid and lasting.

NOTES

Application

Diets that promise to help you lose weight quickly are suspect. They use tricks that make you weigh less, but often have no lasting effect. Overweight people can usually lose one to two pounds a week on a well-balanced program of healthy eating and exercise. That's the wise way to take (and keep) weight off.

The Wrong Way to Lose Weight

This chapter lists three wrong ways to lose weight. Look them up, then explain what's wrong with them.

1. *Diuretics (water pills)* _____

_____

2. *Extra protein* _____

_____

3. *Starvation diets* _____

_____

The Right Way to Lose Weight

By switching to the *Optimal Diet* plus some walking, you can lose one to two pounds a week. That might not get you slim in time for summer, but it is a sensible health-conscious approach to long-term weight management. Read on until you get to page 176; you'll be amazed!

How Fiber Helps

One of the many virtues of fiber is that it acts as a safety mechanism to keep you from overeating. It helps you feel full before you can eat too many calories.

Fiberless foods lack this automatic shutoff. By the time you feel full, you've eaten enough calories for a family of five. Willpower is the only thing that stands between you and obesity—and we all know how effective that is!

Low-Fiber Foods

All animal products lack fiber. That includes meat, chicken, pork, fish, lobster, milk, eggs, and cheese.

In addition, modern food-processing mills take the fiber out of many foods that used to have it. Sugar, white flour, oils, and most packaged foods fall into this category.

Corn oil is a good example of this process. It takes 14 ears of corn to make one tablespoon of oil. Imagine trying to eat 14 ears of corn at one sitting. Impossible! Yet it's easy to sit down and eat several tablespoons of oil in the form of salad dressings and fried foods.

Your Challenge:

Fruits, vegetables, whole grains, and legumes are high in fiber. Eat them in abundance. Start with this low-fat, high-fiber soup. Serve it with hearty whole-wheat bread and a salad. Eat all you want. You'll fill up long before you'll fatten up.

Split-Pea Soup (for six)

1 c	split peas	1/2 tsp	thyme
6 c	water	1	celery stalk, chopped
1 c	onions	1	potato, chopped
1/4 c	barley	1	carrot, chopped
1	bay leaf	1/2 tbs	sweet basil

Add peas, water, onions, barley, and bay leaf to Crockpot and cook until "almost" tender. Add remaining ingredients and cook another 45 to 60 minutes. Add water if necessary. Leftovers can be used as a spread for bread or as a topping on baked potatoes.

Eat whole fruits, with all their fiber, instead of drinking the juice.

DIETS

Quick-fix Traps

You don't need a new "diet"—you need a new dietary lifestyle!

We spend billions of dollars every year on diets and weight-control paraphernalia, yet the results are dismal. For many, permanent, successful weight control is more difficult to achieve than victory over drugs, tobacco, or alcohol.

Would it be better to stop trying? just to stay fat?

Yes, it would be safer to remain obese than to jump from one diet fad to another, lose pounds now, and gain them back later. Research shows that this yo-yo effect gradually depletes important body tissues such as muscle and bone. Eventually it weakens the body so that it becomes more susceptible to disease and less able to shed excess fat.

But isn't it dangerous to remain overweight?

Being fat isn't healthful. Excess weight impairs health and shortens life. As little as 10 to 15 pounds of extra weight produces measurable changes that can lay the foundation for degenerative disease. And for every 10 pounds of overweight, the life span can be shortened by as much as a year.

So what is the answer?

People who are overweight need major revisions in thinking and attitudes. The scenario played out in millions of lives goes something like this: a few weeks on the latest wonder diet; have the jaws wired; take a series of shots or pills; have the stomach stapled; get an intestinal bypass; check into a fat farm. And presto, down goes the weight! Celebration! New clothes!

But within days these people resume their former eating patterns and lifestyle. In a few weeks or months their lost pounds are back, often with a bonus.

Weight-control programs usually fail because they are short-term fixes for long-term problems. It's time to face the reality that obesity can be a serious and life-threatening condition.

OK, I'm convinced. What must I do?

Managing obesity is much more than a dietary problem. Like diabetes, hypertension, alcoholism, or smoking, obesity requires a comprehensive approach to lifestyle changes.

- *First,* you have to have a long-term commitment to better health, a commitment that does not change when binges or other lapses occur. With this kind of commitment you can get up when you fall, start again, and persevere.
- *Second,* you need to identify and change habits that cause obesity. This may be as simple as eliminating soft drinks or cutting back on fats and oils. Or it may require you to restructure your eating patterns and your lifestyle completely.

Changing lifelong habits is among the most difficult things a person can do. For many people the process can be very threatening. Faithful, regular

Surveys reveal that at any one time 40 to 50 percent of Americans between 35 and 59 years old are on a diet.

meetings with a support group greatly increase the chances of success. This kind of team effort is almost a must for those more than 30 pounds overweight, or who have had problems for several years.

- *Third,* attitudes often need radical surgery. Willingness to

change is critically important. Read books, attend seminars, join fitness groups, and make friends with health-minded people. Weight control is not a vanity trip. Keep the focus on improved health, and the weight will take care of itself.

- *Finally,* look for a weight-control plan that is consistent with a lifetime of good health. This will include a low-fat, high-fiber diet, regular exercise, and a physical, mental, and psychological outlook that meets your needs. Weight control should be only part of a full and fulfilling life—not its main preoccupation.

Such a workable life plan is possible. Many have succeeded. Put your heart into it and keep it there.

To Your Good Health!

The dream of many people is a magic pill taken before each meal that will remove all the calories.

In the absence of such a magic pill, we continue to try dozens of diets, spend a fortune on exercise equipment and health club memberships, and even hire trainers who will come to our homes and work out with us.

We read so much about what is good for us and what is bad that the picture has become muddled. Advertising nowadays is so slick that we often don't know what to believe anymore. To help you, here are some hard facts you can depend on. To accomplish weight loss in a healthy way:

- Always have a breakfast. In a hurry? Try a bagel, toast, or dry cereal.
- Carry your lunch to avoid fast food. Stay away from vending machines.
- Go outdoors for a brisk walk during lunch. Join a health club.
- Try new low-fat, easy-to-prepare recipes for dinner.
- Eat before you go to a party at which dietary dangers abound.
- Find a support partner to collaborate in weight and exercise goals.

Begin early in a child's life to shape healthful attitudes toward food. Don't use favorite foods as a bribe or withhold them as punishment. When food is linked to behavior, the food takes on a far greater meaning than it should in a child's life.

NOTES

The 10 Principles of Losing Weight

1. *Think long-term.* Shortcuts and quickie plans never last.
2. *Do it for yourself.* Improving your health and energy are better motivations than a coming class reunion.
3. *Prepare the way.* Don't rush into a diet before you are ready for long-term changes. Keeping a diet journal will help you become more aware of what you eat and why.
4. *Think fruits, grains, legumes, and vegetables.* In the standard American diet more than 50 percent of calories come from fat, sugar, and alcohol.
5. *Control portion sizes.* Use a smaller plate. Serve yourself smaller portions and put away leftovers before you eat. At restaurants, ask for a doggie bag instead of cleaning your plate.
6. *Eat three meals a day.* Eating at regular intervals will not send your body into a deprivation (starvation) mode, which may cause you to eat and binge more.
7. *Maintain your program.* Successful weight-loss managers realize that they are not on a temporary diet—they are starting a permanent new lifestyle.
8. *Exercise.* It's fun and keeps you flexible. Activity is the key to successful weight control, particularly in middle age.
9. *Don't overdo it.* Don't push yourself to the higher end of the target range. A brisk one-hour walk a day is a terrific goal for steady, healthy weight management.
10. *When you think activity, think "play."* Walking the dog, gardening, yardwork, household chores, sports, bicycling, and playing with kids are all productive activities. How do kids exercise? They play! You can have fun too.

Application

Diets are quick-fix traps that don't last. Many people skip from one to the next, losing weight now and gaining it back later. This cycle is discouraging, defeating, and often dangerous. A lifetime commitment to good health practices is the only safe path to permanent weight control.

Take the Long-term Approach

It's virtually impossible to lose weight and keep it off if you don't modify your lifestyle. Diets are a short-term solution to a long-term problem. That is why most dieters regain their lost weight within a year.

Make eating the right foods a permanent part of your daily life. This is the solution to weight control. You can beat the bulge and live a happier, healthier life. Here's how:

Basic Guidelines for Good Eating

Turn to the summary on page 246. You can have fun too. Read each item carefully, imagining how you could incorporate it into your way of living.

Can You Make the Commitment?

Turn inward for a moment. Can you make a long-term commitment to this style of eating? Are you willing to bypass the seductive offers of diets that claim to "melt the pounds off" in favor of a focus on good health?

Take a few minutes to think it through. Then answer the following question: "How do I feel about making a lifelong switch to this way of eating?" Be honest with yourself. Give the part of you that wants to eat only chocolate as much of a voice as the part that prom-

ises never to eat anything "bad" again. Recognize that each voice is an extreme that exists in all of us. Lasting change happens somewhere in the middle, and it does not happen overnight. It is a growth process in which new behaviors and values gradually replace old ones. Now go back to the question and answer it. Use an extra sheet of paper if necessary.

_____

_____

_____

_____

_____

Your Challenge:

Read the *Optimal Diet* outline on page 246. Study the 10 principles until you know them well. Start putting them into practice. The reward is worth every effort.

> The REAL RISK comes when people cut back on fat and load up on sweets and other refined foods and snacks instead of eating more real foods, such as potatoes, rice, fruits, and vegetables.

NOTES
_____

_____

_____

_____

_____

The Carbonated Generation

Americans consume twice as much soda pop as they did 25 years ago—a habit that contributes to obesity, tooth decay, and loss of bone mass. We now average two cans of soda a day for every man, woman, and child in this country.

Aren't soft drinks a good way to help people drink more fluids?

Take one glass of water, add eight to 12 teaspoons of sugar, mix in a dose of chemicals—and you've got a soft drink.

The extra sugar intake from soft drinks produces at least five undesirable side effects:

1. *Unbalanced nutrition.* Most soft drinks contain 120 to 180 calories of sugar, but no needed nutrients.

   A typical sedentary woman requires only about 1,200 to 1,600 total calories a day to maintain optimal weight and good health. Two or three soft drinks can considerably reduce her daily food allotment and thus also her nutrient supply. Over time this imbalance could cause her nutritional status to become marginal.

   The same applies to sedentary men, who may need about 1,800 to 2,400 calories a day.

2. *Extra fat storage.* If the soft drink calories are added to the food calories, the excess will be stored as fat.

Soda pop is the number one source of refined sugar in the U.S. diet, providing the average person with one third of their sugar intake. Teenage boys get 44 percent of their 34 teaspoons of sugar a day from soft drinks; girls, 40 percent of their 24 teaspoons.

3. *Uneven blood sugar.* Sugar calories lack fiber and rapidly enter the bloodstream, raising blood sugar levels and providing a temporary boost of energy. When the blood sugar level goes up, insulin enters the bloodstream to pull the raised blood sugar back down, and energy levels drop. This sequence promotes the cycle of reaching for another, and yet another, soft drink or other sugary snack.

4. *Delayed digestion.* When a sugared drink arrives in a stomach that is processing other food, digestion slows down until the new calories can be handled. An occasional drink probably wouldn't make much difference, but if it happens several times a day it can prolong digestion and stress the stomach.

5. *Acid rebound.* Most beverages, including sodas, increase acid secretion in the stomach. This increase usually occurs after the beverage leaves the stomach, producing a rebound effect.

HOW MANY CALORIES DO YOU DRINK IN A DAY?

Drink	Serving Size	Cal.	Number of Servings	Total Calories
Coffee, cream, and sugar	1 cup	75		
Orange juice	1 cup	110		
Soft drinks, juice, punch	12 oz	140		
Diet soft drinks	12 oz	0		
Nonfat milk	1 cup	90		
Whole milk	1 cup	160		
Milk shake	12 oz	425		
Beer	12 oz	150		
Cocktail	1	150		
Mineral water/Water	12 oz	0		
			Your Grand Total	

No wonder diet drinks have become so popular! Is this a good solution?

Diet drinks solve the sugar problem, but that's not the whole story. Most beverages, sugared or not, contain preservatives, flavorings, colorings, and many other chemicals. Some of these need to be detoxified and eliminated from the body. Some may also irritate sensitive stomach linings.

Many soft drinks, whether diet or not, contain phosphoric acid, a powerful chemical used to etch glass. Americans already consume too much phosphorus, which the body eliminates through the kidneys by combining it with calcium. With today's worries about osteoporosis, the bone-thinning disease, the fact that each phosphorus-containing soft drink takes some calcium from the bones could be a greater risk than many want to take.

What, then, is the safest way to meet body fluid needs?

Water is the perfect beverage. It has no calories, requires no digestion, does not irritate, and is exactly what the body needs to carry on the life processes. How much should we drink? We should drink enough to keep the urine pale—about six to eight glasses of water a day.

Tired? Drink More Water

People by and large know they should down eight glasses of water a day, and most end up getting about that much from water, milk, and juice. But according to a survey by Cornell Medical Center, they also imbibe a daily average of five cups of caffeinated or alcoholic beverages. Both dehydrate the body, leading to fatigue, dry skin, indigestion, and headaches. The solution? For every alcoholic drink and for every cup of coffee or cola, drink an extra glass of water.

SOFT DRINKS

Orange juice may be nutritious, but it's not as good as the original orange. Orange juice, after all, is defibered orange. The whole fruit, when compared to juice, requires less insulin to assimilate, lowers cholesterol more effectively, provides smoother digestion with longer appetite satisfaction, and has fewer calories.

Several soft drink manufacturers encourage feeding soft drinks to toddlers by licensing their logos to makers of baby bottles. Infants and toddlers are four times likelier to be fed soda pop out of these bottles than out of regular baby bottles.

THE EXPANDING SODA BOTTLE

6½ oz.

12 oz.

20 oz.

Bigger serving sizes spur consumption. In the 1950s Coca-Cola was sold as a 6½-ounce bottle. That grew to a 12-ounce can, which was soon augmented by 20-ounce bottles. And now there's the 64-ounce, 600-calorie "Double Gulp"—the Pop Belly Special!

NOTES

Application

North Americans, on average, drink more soft drinks than water. That means they are getting a lot of calories but not much nutrition. Drinking calorie-loaded beverages is one sure recipe for gaining weight. Switch to water—it's the slender person's drink of choice.

An Inventory

What are you drinking? Sometimes it's eye-opening to find out. Listed on page 149 are some popular beverages. How many of each do you drink on a typical day? Then, for each type of beverage, multiply the number consumed by the number of calories. Write this in the Total Calories column. When you're done, add all the totals to get your Grand Total.

Drinking It On

It takes 3,500 excess calories to make a pound of fat. Assuming you eat enough to maintain your weight, how many days would it take you to drink on an extra pound?

You can calculate this by dividing 3,500 by the number of calories you get from beverages each day. For example, if you drank a beer and two coffees, the calculation would be:

Total calories for a beer and two coffees = 300.
3,500/300 = 11.6 days

In other words, it would take just under 12 days to add an extra pound of fat. At that rate you could gain 30 pounds a year just from what you drink!

Now it's your turn. Take your Grand Total from the previous exercise and divide it into 3,500 to see how long it takes you to drink an extra pound's worth of calories. Fill in the blanks below.

Number of days to drink 3,500 calories
3,500 ÷ calories you drink _____ = _____ days

Water Is the Way to Go

If you are serious about controlling your weight, it would be wise to eliminate those sneaky liquid calories. Stop the sodas, lose the liquor, shelve the shakes. Water is what your body needs and craves.

Your Challenge:

Cut calories by drinking more water and fewer high-calorie beverages. If you don't like the taste of tap water, add a twist of lemon or buy bottled water. The more water you drink, the less likely you are to reach for other beverages. That alone will cut calories and help stabilize your weight.

NOTES

NO ENERGY?

You may be dehydrated. Your body needs six to eight glasses of water besides other beverages. In fact, since caffeine pulls water out of your system, every time you have a caffeinated drink you need to back it up with extra water. Keep your body hydrated, and it may chase away that tired feeling.

A Nation of Grazers

Americans spend $13 billion a year on salted snack foods such as potato chips, pork rinds, popcorn, and the like. And we spend at least that much more on sweet snacks.

We need snacks, don't we? I read somewhere that it's difficult to get all the nutrients a person needs without snacks.

That bit of wisdom came out of a study done on children. It holds up only when children don't get nourishing, well-balanced meals, or when they aren't hungry enough at mealtime to eat the calories they need.

Most Americans, children or adults, have no real idea what it's like to be hungry. From birth, kids are fed almost constantly. The habit carries on through the years. We have become a nation of grazers.

But "grazing" is supposed to be a good way to lose weight! You eat a little every hour or so all day. That way you don't get hungry, so you don't overeat.

Actually, the calories gained from snacks and beverages can add up to more calories than some people should eat all day!

Suppose, for instance, you have a midmorning snack of coffee with cream and sugar and a jelly doughnut.

Add a midafternoon snack of a soft drink and a candy bar, plus a late-afternoon snack of a cup of coffee with cream and sugar and three cookies.

Commercials push the idea that we need some kind of energy lift between meals. Yet most snacks are junk food—coffee, colas, cheese, soda pop, popcorn, cookies, salami, milk chocolate, chocolate-chip cookies, chips, crackers, doughnuts, candy bars . . .

Top it off in the evening with a typical TV snack: a soft drink, 10 potato chips, and five cheese crackers. If this sounds familiar, you'd better watch out—all that snacking added some 1,500 calories to your day! Now you know why the old saying is still true: The bigger the snacks, the bigger the slacks. Many people, as a matter of fact, have gained control of their weight simply by cutting out snacking.

But a lot of people can't get through the day without those "pick-me-up" snacks!

That's because they eat refined, fiber-poor, sugar-rich meals, without enough unrefined complex carbohydrates (starches) and fiber. A breakfast of presweetened dry cereal and

orange juice, for instance (or coffee and doughnut), is quickly digested. The sugars rush into the bloodstream, push up the blood sugar, and provide a temporary high.

But it doesn't hold for long, and when the blood sugar drops, there

The bigger the snacks, the bigger the slacks.

is that weak, all-gone feeling that cries to be relieved by a beverage or snack. And the cycle repeats itself.

A breakfast of whole-grain cooked cereal, whole-wheat bread, and a couple whole fresh fruits, on the other hand, will furnish plenty

of steady energy all morning long. A similarly high-complex-carbohydrate, high-fiber lunch will do the same for the afternoon.

Are you saying that we don't need snacks?

The snack habit is just that, a habit. With regular, adequate meals there will be much less need for snacks.

What's more, people have fewer digestive problems when they eat simple meals of mostly high-fiber plant foods and then allow their stomachs to rest for a while. Ideally, meals should be spaced about four to five hours apart.

If you suffer from indigestion, heartburn, irritability, insomnia, mental dullness, gas, or weight gain,

A Snack Study

At a large university a group of students received a breakfast of cereal, toast, fruit, and an egg. Within four hours their stomachs were empty.

A few days later the same students ate the same breakfast, but two hours later were given either a peanut butter sandwich or a piece of pumpkin pie with a glass of milk. Six to nine hours later a part of that breakfast was still in their stomachs.

One person received a little chocolate twice in the morning and twice during the afternoon. Some 13 hours after breakfast, more than half the breakfast was still in the stomach.

CALORIES FROM SNACKS AND BEVERAGES

Midmorning	Coffee with cream and sugar	75
	Jelly doughnut	255
Midafternoon	Soft drink	140
	Candy bar	295
Late Afternoon	Coffee with cream and sugar	75
	Cookies (3)	350
TV Snack	Soft drink	140
	Potato chips (10)	125
	Cheese crackers (5)	90
Calories from snacks and beverages		**1,545**

it could be because of between-meal snacking. A pattern of three meals a day with no snacking could solve many of these problems.

Any suggestions for a "must have a snack" attack?

Drink a big glass of water. It has no calories and requires no digestion. It passes right through, giving everything a good rinse.

If you must have more, eat a piece of fresh fruit or a handful of raw veggies.

The best way to fight off a snack attack, however, is to remember that the calories you save by shunning those snacks will gradually melt off unwanted bulges.

While it may not always be true that once on the lips, forever on the hips, there's no more doubting the fact that the bigger the snacks, the bigger the slacks.

NOTES

The calories you get from snacking can add up to an extra meal—a big one at that. Many people are able to control their weight just by kicking the snack habit. You can too, by eating adequate meals high in unrefined complex carbohydrates and fiber. These meals will provide you with the steady energy you need to make it from one meal to the next.

Warning: Snacking Can Be Hazardous

Stop for a moment and think of the foods you snack on. Do you reach for a juicy apple, or do you unwrap a candy bar? Do you munch raw vegetables, or tear into a sack of chips? Most people opt for high-sugar, high-fat, high-salt goodies to get them from one meal to the next. The extra pounds they wear testify to their devotion.

If you want to lose weight, you must deal with that snack habit. Here are some hints to help you make the change:

Don't Snack for the Wrong Reasons

People snack for many reasons besides hunger. Some people use it as a way to release stress. Others feel guilty taking a break. To them, eating something is a way to legitimize a needed rest.

Do you snack only when you're hungry, or do you use snacks to meet other needs? Think about this, then write down some of your reasons for snacking.

Start With a Good Breakfast

Beating the snack habit begins with a hearty breakfast. It should provide plenty of unrefined complex carbohydrates for lasting energy. Let whole grains, which are high in these carbohydrates, form the core of the meal.

Watch Out for Triggers

Many habits, snacking included, are linked to signals from your environment. For example, you might get the urge for a candy bar whenever you pass that vending machine at work. Or there might be a certain television commercial that makes you want to open a bag of chips. What triggers your urge to snack?

Develop Alternate Behaviors

How do you fight a snack attack? By doing other things to disrupt the pattern. If you are bogged down in your work and need a boost, go for a quick walk to the corner and back. Drink a glass of water rather than the usual soda. If you must eat something, try a piece of fruit or some raw vegetables.

Your Challenge:

Break the night's fast and start your mornings with a hearty breakfast, and skip the midmorning goodies. Together these habits will help you look good and feel better.

Building a Hearty Breakfast

Cereals—cooked cereal, waffles, low-fat granola topped with banana, peaches, berries, etc.

Fresh Whole Fruit—all types, especially citrus and melon

Additional Fruit—fresh or frozen without sugar

Bread—whole-wheat or multigrain bread

Protein—tofu, legumes, or a little nut butter

REMEMBER

Every extra pound shaves off about one month from your life span. Sixty pounds can cost you five years of life!

Walk Out of Obesity

I n America today, fitness is in. Strut your sweat. Lace up your Reeboks. Flaunt your leotards. The majority of Americans, however, are woefully unfit and feeling out of step.

When I hear that a person has to run 10 miles to work off an ice-cream sundae, I feel like—"What's the use!"

There are other choices. You can burn the calories by sleeping for 15 hours or by watching TV for 12 hours. The problem, of course, is that there aren't enough hours in the day to sleep away an ice-cream sundae along with your other meals. That's why exercise is so important. It helps your body burn calories faster.

The body is a motor that runs all the time. The rate at which the body motor idles is called its basal metabolic rate (BMR). The faster the motor runs, the more fuel is used.

However, when fuel supplies are cut (not enough calories consumed), an inner mechanism turns down the body's idling speed. Available fuel now burns more slowly. This function is lifesaving under conditions of starvation, but it defeats the person trying to lose weight.

Can this reaction be prevented?

Activity speeds up the body's metabolic rate. Not only are more calories burned during exercise, but the effect continues for several

We can no longer afford to be complacent about the epidemic of obesity in America. Overweight kills primarily by promoting heart disease, stroke, and many cancers. Marked obesity may increase the risk of diabetes in adults by 10 times and contribute heavily to chronic disease and disability.

—Harvard University Nurses' Health Study

hours. That's why most people feel more energetic when they exercise. The BMR (basal metabolic rate) of the body reflects this. A regular exercise program promotes weight loss by pepping up the metabolism—burning calories faster.

How many calories do I need a day?

Multiplying your ideal weight by 10 approximates the daily calories you would need to maintain the status quo if you are inactive—this is your BMR. Most people use an additional 30 percent of their BMR calories for activity calories. Added together, this figure represents the number of calories you need to eat every day to maintain your weight.

If you're fairly sedentary and weigh 150 pounds, for example, your BMR needs would be 1,500 calories, and your activity calories would be 450, for a total of 1,950 calories.

To lose weight, you need to reduce this number of calories (eat less) or increase the number of calories used (exercise more). When you develop a negative energy balance, you force your body to burn its reserve fuel—the fat.

Doesn't muscle tissue turn into fat as a person gets older?

Muscle tissue does not turn to fat. It is physiologically impossible for this to happen.

Muscles are the body's furnace—that's where fat is burned. That's why men seem able to eat more and yet lose weight faster than women.

When people become less active, however, their muscles shrink and their BMR slows down. Eating habits often are not adjusted to this lessened activity, so as excess calories accumulate, the body stores the fat in numerous places, including the spaces around the muscle fibers.

An important point to understand is that the muscles burn fat. When more muscle tissue is present, fat will burn faster and more efficiently. On the other hand, lack of exercise and a "starvation weight-loss regimen" will cause the body to lose muscle. If this situation persists for a long time,

it may become almost impossible to lose further weight.

Is 30 minutes of exercise, three times a week, enough?

The best exercise program for fit people is actually done daily for 30 minutes and alternates between aerobic activity and strength training (weights, calisthenics). But people who need to lose weight must aim higher. Do an hour a day.

What is the best time to exercise?

Anytime. Do it whenever you can squeeze in some time. Or better yet: schedule your exercise. Make it part of your daily lifestyle. Some people prefer to do it first thing in the morning. Then it's done. You feel good. And you are likely to eat less and you'll stimulate your metabolism to burn more calories.

What is the best exercise?

The safest and best exercise is walking; aim for 10,000 a day! Swimming is a close second best. People with higher levels of fitness may choose more strenuous exercises.

Start slowly with what you can do.

Overweight Kids

Many overweight children already have higher blood pressure, insulin, lipid, and "bad cholesterol" levels that make them much more susceptible to disease. Part of that has to do with less exercise.

In 1930 only 7 percent of children were bussed to school. Today more than 50 percent are bussed, and the rest are chauffeured by a parent.

Exercise for Vigor

"Action is a law of our being. Every organ of the body has its appointed work, upon the performance of which its development and strength depend. The normal action of all the organs gives strength and vigor, while the tendency of disuse is toward decay and death."

—Ellen G. White,
The Ministry of Healing

Walking has some major advantages over most other fitness activities:

- few injuries
- doesn't require "stuff"—no wrist pads, goggles, knee pads, helmets, gloves, or poles.
- minimal cost—just the price of a pair of good walking shoes.

Menopause?

Active women are less prone to menopausal symptoms such as hot flashes, anxiety, depression, and sleeplessness.

How fast you go isn't the most important thing. What counts is the total distance covered and the duration of the activity. Some people must start with only five minutes at a time several times a day. A person who walks five minutes, carrying 50 pounds of extra weight, will burn more calories than a person carrying only 20 extra pounds who walks the same distance.

If you want to get in shape, put your best foot forward, begin to walk your way out of obesity, and keep going for a lifetime!

NOTES

A regular exercise program helps you lose weight by boosting your metabolism and strengthening your muscles. It also increases your energy and endurance and lifts your spirits. Exercise is a high-yield investment.

Important Information

Read the last two pages of this chapter; then answer these questions:

1. How much time a day should an overweight person spend exercising?
2. What is the safest and best exercise?

The answers to these questions are important because together they make up the second element of an effective weight-loss program: exercise.

Fortunately, this program can be gentle. You don't need to pump iron or run marathons. Set a goal—to achieve 10,000 steps a day. Then get yourself some comfortable walking shoes and step out the front door. . . .

No Time to Exercise

Everyone is rushed these days. Even kids and retirees have full calendars. Squeezing in a half hour of exercise every day can seem like an impossible dream.

Many busy people get their exercise out of the way by getting up a little earlier. Some walk during their lunch hour or at break times. Others like to unwind by walking in the evening after work. Be creative, and you will find that there is always time for a high-priority activity such as exercise.

There Will Be Days

Of course there will be some days you can't complete your whole exercise routine. When that happens, shoot for a shorter walk. A jaunt to the end of the street or around the house is better than no exercise at all.

Don't strive for perfection and then give up when you don't achieve it. Persistence is far more valuable than perfection when it comes to building a healthful lifestyle.

What are some ways you can fit a walk into your day? Write down your ideas in the space below.

_____

_____

_____

_____

No Pain, No Gain?

Maybe you have heard coaches and other "exercise people" say, "No pain, no gain." Forget that advice. Walking can provide the physical activity you need and boost your metabolism. Exercise doesn't have to hurt to be good for you.

Share It With a Friend

One of the best things about walking is you don't need to do it alone. Walking with others encourages communication. Many couples find it strengthens their relationship, and friends enjoy a companionship that makes the miles fly by.

Your Challenge:

Make walking a part of each day. Aim for 10,000 steps a day. Start with just 10 minutes a day, and work up from there. When combined with a proper diet, walking is an effective way to keep your weight under control. But also check with the local gym or YMCA to enroll in a strength and flexibility training program to round out your overall fitness.

> People who regularly walk one and a half to three miles a day have less heart disease, less cancer, less diabetes, less obesity, and fewer colds.

Building Caloric Bombs

We often take healthful, nutritious foods and turn them into caloric bombs. It's easy. It's insidious. And we do it without thinking.

Take an apple, for instance. It has vitamins, minerals, fiber, and only 70 calories. If we ate apples as they came from the tree, we'd have no problem. But we love to douse them with sugar and make applesauce—doubling the calories. Or we squeeze out the juice, removing most of the fiber and concentrating the calories. Even more popular is apple pie, an American special ranked along with motherhood, the flag, and baseball. It's also a nutritional disaster—one slice à la mode can easily pack 500 calories.

I could eat a lot of apples for that!

That's the point. You would have to eat at least six apples to reach that caloric level. And you know you wouldn't do that. You'd feel full after two or three.

Or take the potato. By itself the lowly spud is a wonderfully nutritious food. How good is it? Well, a few years ago a scientist tried an experiment. He ate nothing but potatoes for a whole year. Surprisingly, he remained in good health with plenty of energy.

But look at the way we eat potatoes today. A seven-ounce potato, by itself, contains about 120 calories. But who eats a plain

Socializing with others is an important part of a healthy lifestyle. Just remember—you don't have to eat everything offered.

potato? Look on the next page to see some of the ways we dress it up.

And that's just the tip of the iceberg. Fresh salads are doused with oily dressings. Most of our fruit goes into juices or pies, or is canned in heavy syrup. Even when we cook fresh vegetables we usually butter them, or add a sauce, which can double and triple the calories. No wonder people have weight problems!

How can we go about reversing this trend?

The solutions are relatively simple. Food preferences, after all, are not in-born; they are learned and cultivated. They can be changed. Substituting a good habit and repeating it over and over with persistence and determination will do the trick.

You can begin by eating more natural foods that have been simply prepared. This includes whole-grain products such as whole-wheat bread, whole-grain cereals, rice, and pasta. It also includes fresh vegetables of all kinds. Tubers such as potatoes and yams, and legumes, such as beans, peas, and lentils, are excellent choices.

Indulge yourself with fruit. Whenever possible, eat fresh, whole fruit without added sugar. Peeling and eating an orange, for example, instead of drinking the juice, gives you more food value and fiber, and it fills you up with fewer calories.

When food is eaten as grown, it is full of fiber and quite low in calories. By leaving those caloric bombs alone, at least most of the time, you can actually eat a larger quantity of food, feel full and satisfied, and still lose weight.

> ## Eliminating the loved and familiar requires commitment and fortitude.

More than 4,000 times every day someone in the United States has a heart attack. Heart disease, cancer, hypertension, obesity, and diabetes are epidemic in America as they are in other industrialized countries, where people can afford diets rich in meat, fish, poultry, and eggs, and loaded with refined, engineered foods high in sugar, fat, and salt.

FOOD REFINEMENT CONCENTRATES CALORIES AND CHANGES CALORIC DENSITY

80 Calories

480 Calories

	Calories
Baked Potato	**120**
With Sour Cream and Butter	390
Hash Browns	450
French Fries	460
Potato Chips	1,000
Pringles	1,120

70 Calories

370 Calories

Valentine choco-lates are always one of the great mysteries of life: How can one pound in the shape of a heart add two pounds in the shape of your bottom?

Eliminating the loved and familiar requires commitment and fortitude.

Almost as Big as the Pentagon —but With Cheese!

"All told, Americans eat 90 acres of pizza every day."
—*American Health*

IT'S TIME TO MAKE A HEALTHY DIFFERENCE

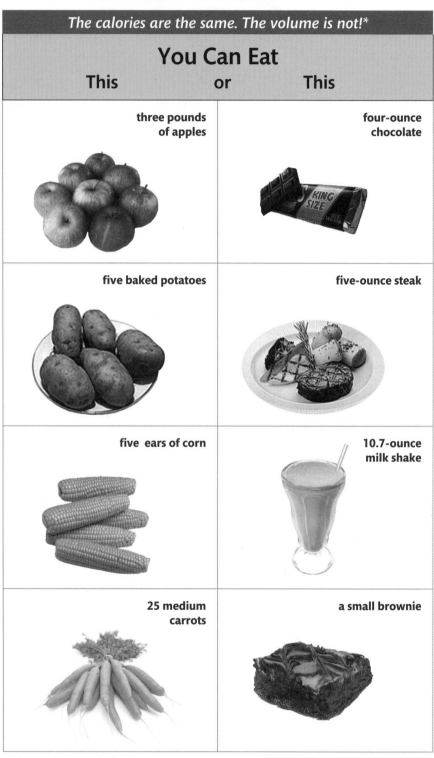

*The calories are the same. The volume is not!**	
You Can Eat	
This or	**This**
three pounds of apples	four-ounce chocolate
five baked potatoes	five-ounce steak
five ears of corn	10.7-ounce milk shake
25 medium carrots	a small brownie

*approximate equivalents

Food preferences are not inborn. They are learned and cultivated.

Application

We are not born with food preferences; they are habits we develop. By re-educating ourselves to avoid "caloric bombs" and to enjoy more natural, low-fat foods, we can eat more, feel full, and still lose weight.

How many calories do you need?

How many calories can you eat before your body begins storing the excess as fat? To find out, start by calculating how many calories your body needs to keep you alive over a 24-hour period.

Your basal metabolic rate (BMR for short) is the rate at which your body would burn calories if you decided to stay in bed all day. You can estimate your BMR calories by multiplying your ideal weight by 10.

BMR Calories Per Day

Ideal Weight _____ x 10 = _____ Calories

Now, if you don't have an exercise program or engage in heavy labor, you will need an additional 30 percent of your BMR calories to cover your activity calories. For example, if your BMR calories totaled 1,500, you would need an additional 450 calories to cover your activity calories. Calculate your activity calories by multiplying your BMR calories by 0.3.

Daily Activity Calories

BMR Calories _____ x 0.3 = _____ Calories

The final step is to add your BMR and activity calories to get the number of calories you burn in a day. If you eat more than this amount, your body will deposit the excess calories as fat. If you eat less, your body uses fat from its stores, and you lose weight.

Calories You Burn Daily

BMR Cal. _____ + Activity Cal. _____ = _____ Cal.

A Caloric Bomb Disaster

It would be hard to exceed your calorie limit on the Optimal Diet because whole foods are high in fiber and low in fat. But when you start adding fat, watch out! Look what happens to this meal:

Food	Cal.	Added Fat	Cal.	Total Cal.
Lettuce and Tomato Salad	40 +	Roquefort Dressing	160	200
Whole-Wheat Bread	65 +	Butter	70	135
Broccoli (½ c)	35 +	Cheese Sauce	130	165
Vegetarian Entrée or Broiled Fish (6½ oz)	220 +	Tartar Sauce	100	320
Baked Potato With Salsa	135 +	Butter and Sour Cream	180	315
Skim Milk (1 gal)	90	Whole Milk		160
Baked Apple With Date and Walnut	100	Apple Pie à la mode (⅙)		480
Total Calories	**685**	**Total Calories**		**1,775**

Your Challenge:

Avoid "caloric bombs." Work to reduce the oils, butters, dressings, and gravies you add to your food. It's time to shift the scales in your favor!

NOTES

_____

_____

_____

_____

_____

Getting Fatter Faster

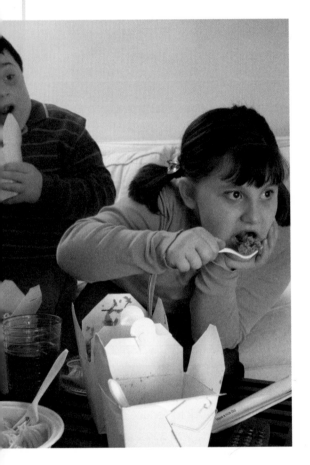

American children are now getting fatter faster than ever. Six million youngsters aged 5 to 11 now have serious weight problems: they are classified as *obese*. That's every 5th child. The number of *super-fat* children has tripled over the past 25 years. If these trends continue, every third child and teenager will be obese by 2030.

That's hard to believe. Isn't our culture more health-conscious now? Aren't fitness clubs booming?

Physical fitness is a trend among adults, not children. It's grown-ups who are out running, walking, jogging, and joining fitness clubs and aerobic classes. It's the older people who are flocking to wellness lectures and examining menus at restaurants for healthier and leaner foods.

But don't schools have health courses, physical education, and sports activities?

Yes, but because of budget cuts, overcrowding, and teacher shortages, many schools have had to cut back on these programs in recent years. In some cases they've eliminated physical education courses and requirements altogether. Health classes are often unpopular with students, and relatively few youngsters qualify for team positions in school-sponsored sports.

Isn't obesity in children mostly inherited?

Genes do play a role in a person's weight, but they aren't the whole answer. Environment plays a critically important role—as shown by the fact that the percentage of obese Americans has increased steadily over the past 40 years. Our gene pool can't change that fast!

We now have an environment that supports obesity. Once upon

Today's children average 5 to 8 hours a day watching television, playing computer games, or texting! Our entire culture promotes less physical activity and more eating.

a time children raced home from school to change clothes and go outside to play. They climbed trees, rode bicycles, skated, played games, and dribbled basketballs. Today's children average five to eight hours a day watching television or playing computer games or texting! Our entire culture promotes less physical activity and more eating.

What are the chances of a fat child becoming a fat adult?

About 80 percent of overweight teenagers will remain overweight as adults. The marked increase in adolescent obesity will have serious consequences in the future. And dieting is not the answer.

Some 80 percent of American girls begin a regular cycle of dieting by the time they are just 11 years old, according to William Rader, M.D.

Does obesity produce disease in childhood?

Being overweight predisposes a child to heart disease, gallstones, adult-onset diabetes, hypertension, cancer, and full-blown obesity later in life. Obese children have more or-

thopedic problems and upper-respiratory diseases. And that is only one side of the story. They often suffer major social and psychological problems. The rapid increase of serious depression, eating disorders, drug use, suicide, and violence among teenagers is frightening.

What can be done about this growing problem?

The major causes of obesity in children are the same as for adults—a sedentary lifestyle, TV viewing, the snack and soda habit, and the popularity and availability of highly processed and concentrated foods. Many major medical centers are developing weight-control programs for children that involve the whole

Teen Weight Trends: Going the Wrong Way!

By age group, 20 percent of kids, 6-11 years of age, are *obese*. For kids ages 12-19 it's 18%. . . . And when it comes to *overweight*, 32% of kids 2-19 years of age are too heavy. Many parents do not perceive the problem, and more than 80 percent believe that their child is physically fit.

Thousands of school-age children have serious weight problems that affect their health, their ability to perform, and their peer acceptance.

To these children and their families, obesity is a curse. To do nothing is to sentence them to a possible lifetime of social misery, rejection, and a significantly higher risk of developing early major health problems (see next page).

Monitor your child's emotional life. Some children eat when they feel nervous or unhappy; others when they are alone or neglected. Problems may start during a divorce. Look for unmet emotional needs. ABOVE ALL—make your kids feel loved, unconditionally.

Is Your Child in Crisis?

Saving the child just might save the family.

Increasingly, Type II (adult-onset) diabetes is turning up in children, and health experts fear an impending health crisis. So far, all studies have pointed to obesity as a factor.

Pre-school children who are obese are likely to continue to be obese as adolescents and adults. Cardiovascular risk factors, such as elevated levels of cholesterol, triglycerides, insulin and blood pressure have been identified in 60% of obese children at the age of 5 to 7 years.

Compared with healthy children, the health-related quality of life of children who are obese is so poor that it is similar to that of children with cancer.

family. Proper eating and lifestyle habits are a family affair, and a youngster especially needs the support of the family. Even when the rest of the family is not overweight, everyone benefits from a healthier way of life.

Seven Secrets for Fat-proofing Your Child

Clinical psychologists and pediatricians feel that nearly all obesity in children could be prevented if children were taught the following sensible basic habits early, before they have free access to food and become addicted to TV:

1. Three meals a day at regular times with lots of _ whole grains, legumes, fresh fruit, and vegetables.
2. Cupboard control—get rid of tempting junk foods. Offer fruit and fresh veggies for snacks.
3. Plenty of water. Limit sodas, juices, and other beverages.
4. At least an hour of active exercise daily, preferably outdoors.
5. Regular, quiet study and reading times to replace the hours spent watching TV, or playing computer games.
6. Plenty of rest. Many children are chronically tired. Put them to bed early enough so they awaken _ naturally, in time for a healthy breakfast.
7. A wide range of interests—library visits, music lessons, arts and crafts, family outings, etc.

NOTES

Hours of television, video games, the Internet, and the easy availability of high-calorie snacks are creating a generation of super-fat children. Their obesity predisposes them to a host of lifestyle related illnesses, and has been linked to serious psychological problems. Families can help these children by adopting proper eating and lifestyle habits. Good health is a family affair.

Not-So-Little Jimmy

Jimmy is overweight for an 11-year-old. The heaviest child in his class, he is often teased by the other children. Because he sees himself as slow and awkward, he resists participating in physical education and after-school sports programs. Instead Jimmy spends his afternoons at home watching television, playing video games, and snacking on pop, chips, and other goodies.

June and George, Jimmy's parents, are learning how lifestyle affects health and well-being. They're making efforts to change their own lifestyle, and also want to help their son. After some discussion, they have come up with three strategies.

1. *Lead by Example*

   Since children learn by example, June and George committed themselves to being better role models. They decided that this means regular exercise and no snacking for either of them.

   Could you be a better role model for your children and others in your family? What are some specific things you could do?

2. *Create a Supportive Home Environment*

   To help Jimmy control his snacking, his parents stopped buying soft drinks, chips, and cookies. They replaced these high-calorie temptations with good old-fashioned fruits and vegetables. Television watching and video games were also limited.

Our environment strongly influences what we eat and how we live. Does your home environment help you achieve your lifestyle goals? What could you do to make it better?

_____

_____

_____

_____

3. *Involve Family Members*

   Jimmy was not silent as his life was rearranged, but his howls of protest were tempered by including him in the process. June and George explained the reasons for the changes. They also listened attentively to Jimmy's concerns. Together the three of them chose new recipes to try. In the evening Jimmy rode his bike while his parents walked or jogged. The changes were difficult at first, but after a time they became routine, and eventually they actually became fun.

   People tend to resist changes in those close to them. By explaining why you are making changes and enlisting the aid of others, you can turn resistance into support. How could you involve your children in the lifestyle changes you are making?

Your Challenge:

Use the ideas you came up with in this unit to make your home a place in which good eating habits can flourish. Involve your family in the changes.

NOTES _____

_____

The Right Weight Debate

'm not obese," said one comedian. "I'm just short for my weight!" Whether short or tall, few people are happy about what they weigh.

How can I tell if I'm FIT or FAT?

A person's weight is a highly individual thing, but here are some guidelines. *Obese*, by definition, means being 20 percent or more above one's ideal weight. A person with an ideal weight of 120 pounds would be obese at 144 pounds or more. *Overweight*, on the other hand, usually means being 10 to 19 percent above one's ideal weight. Our hypothetical person with an ideal weight of 120 pounds would be overweight at 132 to 143 pounds.

How is your "ideal" weight determined?

Ideal weight can be set in different ways. One way is to look at the records of large life insurance companies. They are very interested in finding predictors of longevity because it affects the way they structure their premiums. They have discovered that certain ideal weight-to-height relationships correlate well with optimum life expectancy. The massive actuarial data of the Metropolitan Life Insurance Company formed the basis of its gender-specific Table of Ideal Weight, based on height and bone size.

How is bone size calculated?

Although most people have a pretty good idea of their frame size, wrist (and sometimes ankle) measurements provide a more reliable method. In general, a woman's wrist measurement of five and a

> "By stupid decisions a man ruins his life;
> then he gets angry at God."
> —Proverbs 19:3, Clear Word

quarter inches or less is considered small-boned, between five and a quarter to six inches is medium, and over six inches is large. For men, anything under six inches is small and anything over seven inches is large.

Is there a simpler way to calculate ideal weight?

Here is a time-honored rule of thumb:

- For men—allow 100 pounds for five feet of height. For each additional inch, add six pounds. The ideal weight for a five-foot-ten-inch man would therefore be 160 pounds.
- For women—allow 106 pounds for five feet of height, but add five pounds for each additional inch. For a five-foot-five-inch woman, that comes to 131 pounds. Large-boned men and women can add 5 percent to these figures. Small-boned can subtract 5 percent.

Some athletes I know would flunk that test!

That's right, and that's why it's only a rule of thumb. Football play-

IDEAL WEIGHTS FOR ADULTS BY BODY FRAME
Metropolitan Life Insurance Height/Weight Table (1959)* (weight in lbs.)†

Men				Women			
Height (No Shoes)	Small Frame	Medium Frame	Large Frame	Height (No Shoes)	Small Frame	Medium Frame	Large Frame
5'2"	115-123	121-133	129-144	4'10"	96-104	101-113	109-125
4"	121-129	127-139	135-152	5'0"	102-110	107-119	115-131
6"	128-137	134-147	142-161	2"	108-116	113-126	121-138
8"	136-145	142-156	151-170	4"	114-123	120-135	129-146
10"	144-154	150-165	159-179	6"	122-131	128-143	137-154
6'0"	152-162	158-175	168-189	8"	130-140	136-151	145-163
2"	160-171	167-185	178-199	10"	138-148	144-159	153-173
4"	168-179	177-195	187-209	6'0"	148-158	154-169	163-183

*Many established researchers consider the 1959 table of the Metropolitan Life Insurance Company more consistent with good health than revised tables with higher values.

†Includes one pound for ordinary indoor clothing.

ers, for instance, have more muscle and greater muscle density than the average person. At the same time they carry very little fat. For this reason, the most accurate way to measure body fat is through hydrostatic (underwater) weighing. Fat is buoyant and weighs less under water. This difference allows for calculations of what percentage of a person's body is composed of fat.

One football player consistently weighed in over his maximum allowable weight. He just couldn't lose. Someone finally weighed him under water and found his body fat to be only 5 percent! (10 to 15 percent of body weight as fat is considered excellednt. For women, 15 to 20 percent.)

Where can I get weighed under water?

Look for places that advertise health screening tests. Some of them have tanks of water for this purpose. Others use swimming

Profile of an Overweight Person

- Breakfast skimper
- Takes big bites; eats too fast
- Doesn't drink enough water
- Gets little, if any, exercise
- Uses salt freely
- Likes caffeinated drinks
- Is a nibbler—constantly eating
- Eats mostly refined foods—white breads, white rice, juices, candies, ice cream, etc.

Besides a shortened life span, obese people are at higher risk for painful heel syndrome, stress fractures of the pelvis, and osteoarthritis of the hips and knees. Death and taxes are both inevitable, but ending life as a cripple is not inevitable. Lose that weight now!

Whether we are obese or not still depends on the relationship between the number of calories we eat and the energy we burn.

pools. But it's an inconvenient and complicated process.

A simpler, more practical test is the pinch test. Trained health professionals use calipers to measure the thickness of skin folds at different places on the body. With the proper tables they can then calculate body fat percentages with fair accuracy.

You can do a simplified pinch test yourself. Reach over to your left side, just below the last rib, and pull the skin and fat away from the underlying muscle. Hold it between your thumb and index finger and squeeze. If the space between your thumb and finger is more than three fourths of an inch, you're in trouble!

Obesity can be dangerous. Disease, disability and premature death follow in its train. Next to lowering your cholesterol and quitting smoking, attaining and maintaining an ideal weight is the greatest favor you can do for yourself.

NOTES

Knowing your ideal weight is important. Studies show that people who remain near this target live longer, healthier lives. Find out how close (or far) you are from your ideal weight.

Tale of the Scale

The bathroom scale tells the story of our eating and exercise habits. It can also, for better or worse, predict our health in coming years.

How do you rate? Complete this easy exercise to find out. Before you begin, you will need to know your weight. Also have a calculator handy for calculating percentages.

Calculating Your Ideal Weight

For Men:

1. How many inches over five feet are you? _____
2. Multiply that number by six. _____
3. Add 100 to get your ideal weight. _____

For Women:

1. How many inches over five feet are you? _____
2. Multiply that number by five. _____
3. Add 106 to get your ideal weight. _____

For Women and Men:

Large-boned men and women should multiply their ideal weight by 1.05 to get an ideal weight adjusted for their build. Small-boned persons multiply by 0.95.

Normal Weight

Multiply your ideal weight by 1.09 = _____

If your weight is below this number, you are in the safe range. Regular exercise and a healthy diet will boost your energy and endurance while keeping your weight stable.

Overweight

Multiply your ideal weight by 1.20 = _____

If your weight is below this number but above normal weight, you are classified as overweight. Your weight has reached a level that can affect your health and self-image. It is important to take action now to get your weight under control. Make the *Optimal Diet* and daily exercise a priority.

Obesity

If your weight takes you past overweight, then stop! You are in danger and need to take immediate action. Don't let anything stand between you and daily exercise. Learn to cook healthy meals and put the principles learned in the previous seven chapters into action. If you change your lifestyle now, you can feel years younger and enjoy a longer, healthier life.

CLINICAL WEIGHT DEFINITIONS

	Ideal Weight		
-10%	0	+10%	+20%
Underweight	Normal	Overweight	Obesity

Your Challenge:

A support network can keep you going when you feel like giving up. Find someone else interested in losing weight. Working together will make reaching your goals twice as easy—and twice as enjoyable. Also, graph your weight periodically and then post the record to keep you motivated.

NOTES

_____

_____

_____

_____

_____

Jump-start Your Day

It will boost your energy, increase your attention span, and help you lose weight—and it's legal! What is it? A good breakfast.

Many people can't face food when they crawl out of bed. A quick cup of coffee is a standard adult breakfast. An increasing number of children arrive at school having eaten nothing at all.

Why bother with breakfast?

A group of scientists spent 10 years studying the effects of different kinds of breakfasts versus no breakfast at all on people of different ages.

A good breakfast, they concluded, can help both children and adults be less irritable, more efficient, and more energetic. Breakfast helped children score higher on tests written before the noon recess. The steady influx of energy apparently stabilized glucose levels in the brain, improving mental function and attention span.

Other studies have even linked healthy breakfasts with less chronic disease, increased longevity, and better health.

A good breakfast, by the way, is one that provides at least one third of the day's calories. Start your day with a whole-grain cereal, whole-grain bread, and a couple whole, fresh fruits, and you'll find that your energy level stays high throughout the morning.

What's wrong with orange juice and a Danish?

You need something with more fiber in it. Although fiber isn't digested by the body, it does absorb water as it moves through the stomach and intestines. The resulting spongy mass acts as a gentle barrier to the food particles suspended in it so that they are not absorbed too quickly.

On the other hand, fiberless foods, especially sugared foods and drinks, quickly pass into the bloodstream, and cause blood sugar levels to rise and fall rapidly. No wonder energy and efficiency levels drop off in the later morning hours—little or no fiber-containing foods were eaten at breakfast!

But I'm not hungry until midmorning!

Probably the biggest reason people feel that way is that they eat a large meal in the evening. (TV snacks don't help either!) When they go to bed, their stomachs are still busy digesting all that food. Since digestion goes into a "slower gear" during sleep, sometimes food is still in the stomach in the morning. But the stomach needs rest too. An exhausted stomach does not feel like taking on a big breakfast.

The solution?

- Eat a light supper at least four hours before bedtime, or even skip supper a few times.
- Eat or drink nothing but water or fruit between supper and bedtime.

If you do these two things, you'll be ready to break the fast of the long night.

Won't skipping breakfast help me lose weight?

Surprisingly, no. The Iowa Breakfast Studies demonstrated that the omission of breakfast does not have an advantage in weight reduction. It's actually a disadvantage because those who omit breakfast accentuate their hunger and eat more snacks and food the rest of the day to make up for the lack. They also suffer a significant loss of efficiency in the late-morning hours.

> "I've yet to meet an overweight person who doesn't skip breakfast and snack at night."
>
> —Pat Harper, R.D., American Dietetic Association

But I don't have time to eat breakfast.

Many people are in the habit of staying up late, then sleeping in as long as they can in the morning. Although a few people work more efficiently at night, most don't fit that timetable.

Try going to bed early enough so that you can wake up in the morning feeling refreshed and with time to spare. Begin the day by drinking a glass or two of water to rinse and freshen your stomach. Pull on your gym clothes and get some active exercise, such as a brisk walk. Shower and dress for the day. Then fix and eat a hot breakfast.

This works with children, too. Put them to bed early enough so that they wake up in time to join the family around the breakfast table.

A good breakfast boosts your energy, increases your attention span, and heightens your sense of well-being. You'll be less apt to cheat on your diet by snacking. And you'll be in better control of your emotions.

What a great way to start your day!

How to Pick a Cereal

It's tough to pick a cereal these days. Do you go for fiber, or the least fat and sugar? Whole grains, or more vitamins? Or what the kids demand?

At $4.50 a pound, many cereals cost as much as or more than a pound of cheese, chicken breasts, or sirloin steak. That's because 55 percent of the price goes into marketing and profits—twice as much as the average for other foods.

- Be wary of names and claims. You can trust claims about nutrients, low-fat and high-fiber. But

Sugar in the Morning?

You bet. Millions of us start the day with dessert, whether it's frosted Pop-Tarts, marshmallow-laden cereal, chocolate yogurt, or a muffin the size of a small TV. Then we spend the next 14 hours chugging more sweets, from a midmorning Danish to a vanilla shake at lunch to cookies after dinner. Meanwhile, soft drinks rise around us like floodwaters: we're swigging 54 gallons a year per man, woman, and child!

Food Is Fuel

The brain cells have no stored blood sugar—no energy stores. A lot of people are needlessly fatigued because they're not eating early in the day. They skip breakfast.

BREAKFAST CHOICES

	Calories	Fat (g)	Salt (mg)	Chol. (mg)
Standard American Diet				
Bacon (3 sl)	129	12	574	60
Scrambled Eggs (3)	330	24	1,230	675
Hash Browns (1 c)	355	18	3,265	0
Danish Roll (1)	274	15	595	35
Hot Cocoa (1 c)	213	9	295	25
Orange Juice (1 c)	120	0	6	0
Total	**1,421**	**78**	**5,965**	**795**
The Optimal Diet				
7-Grain Cereal (1 c)	159	1	400	0
Banana (1)	95	0	3	0
NF Milk (1 c)	88	0	318	0
Grapefruit (1/2)	66	0	5	0
Tofu (1 c)	118	7	1,233	0
H. Browns, no oil (1 c)	101	0	22	0
W. W. Bread (1 sl)	61	1	330	0
Total	**688**	**9**	**2,311**	**0**

Honey Nut Cheerios, for example, has more sugar than honey and more salt than nuts. Check the ingredient list. If there is less fruit than sugar, skip it!

- Look for whole grains. Check ingredients to make sure the wheat and oats are "whole" or "rolled" and the rice is brown. Bran is also good.
- Check the fiber. Cancer experts advise up to 40 grams a day (most Americans get only 10 grams). This means: eat lots of whole grains, along with fruit, beans, and vegetables. Look for at least 10 grams of fiber *per meal,* and 15 grams if you are constipated.
- Minimize sugar. It doesn't matter if it's honey, brown sugar, corn syrup, or fruit juice. They all have the same problems. Look for cereals with no more than five grams of added sugar per serving.
- Limit sodium. Look for the least amount of sodium.

- Watch out for fat traps. Most cereals are low in fat, but beware of granola and muesli. Stick to cereals with no more than three grams of fat per serving. Why not try a seven-grain cereal? You can find it in most supermarkets. Pour it into your Crockpot at night. Add enough water. Turn it on, and while you're sleeping your Crockpot is working. You wake up, and a piping-hot delicious breakfast cereal is waiting for you. Just add some fresh fruit, a few raisins or dates, and some milk substitute, such as rice milk or soy milk, and you're purring. You started your day right. You're off and running!

NOTES

Application

A good breakfast boosts your energy, increases your attention span, and heightens your sense of well-being. Studies have now linked healthy breakfasts to less chronic disease, longer life, and better health.

Make the Most of Your Day

Many studies have emphasized the importance of breakfast. If you want to make the most of your day, fuel your body early with the right stuff. The following questions will help you examine your morning eating habits.

The Breakfast Quiz

1. Do you skip breakfast often? Mom was right: Breakfast really is the most important meal of the day. If you skip breakfast, you are starting the day at a disadvantage.

2. Do you get up in time to eat a good breakfast? If not, how could you change your routine to give yourself time for a nutritious morning meal?

   _____

   _____

3. Are you hungry in the morning, or is your appetite a late riser? The preceding pages offer two solutions to this problem. What are they?

   _____

   _____

4. Is your usual breakfast high in fiber from whole fruits and grains? The fiber and complex carbohydrates in whole foods provide a steady release of energy that most processed breakfast foods lack. It will keep you going strong all morning.

5. Is your breakfast high in fat and cholesterol? A traditional breakfast of eggs and sausage can be the most deadly meal of the day. Breakfast meats are loaded with fats, cholesterol, and salt. Egg yolks can send your cholesterol skyrocketing. The sausage-and-egg breakfast needs to go the way of the dinosaur if you want to avoid early extinction.

Based on what you have learned, how can you improve the quality of your breakfasts?

   _____

   _____

   _____

Your Challenge:

Make eating a good breakfast a priority. Note any changes in your energy level and productivity. Here is a recipe to help get you started.

Cashew Oat Waffles

Blenderize the following ingredients until smooth. Bake in a preheated waffle iron for 10-12 minutes:

- 1½ c regular rolled oats
- 2 c water
- ⅓ c raw cashews
- ½ tsp salt

Top with mashed bananas, fresh or frozen berries, applesauce, or crushed pineapple.

NOTES ....

....

....

....

Eat More, Weigh Less!

Two out of three adults in the United States are now overweight or obese. Despite 20 years of increasingly sophisticated diets, the average person is now 17 pounds heavier.

That sounds pretty grim. Is there a brighter side?

Actually, there's a Mr. or Ms. Goodweight inside each one of us—it may just be stuck behind layers of discouragement, bulges of overindulgence, and mounds of misconceptions. We need to locate that special person inside and begin restoring the health, energy, and self-confidence that's been buried far too long.

How do you do that?

By finding a lifestyle that maintains health, increases energy, lowers the risk of disease, reduces food bills, and allows people to eat as much as they want and still lose weight without feeling hungry.

Surely that's an impossible dream!

Not really. Obesity occurs when calories eaten exceed the calories used by the body for physical activity and maintenance of its functions. These leftover calories are stored as fat. By the time 3,500 extra calories have accumulated, one pound of fat will have been deposited.

Adding an extra pat of butter (100 calories) to the daily diet will total up to 10 extra pounds of body fat in one year! On the other hand, omitting dessert (500 calories) for seven days will remove one pound of body fat.

The secret of success lies in finding a way to eat fewer calories instead of eating less food.

That sounds like a contradiction!

Today's world is full of contradictions. Popular magazines and TV screens brim with beautiful, slender people—and with full-color ads of rich, fattening foods. Supermarkets offer 25,000 slickly packaged calorie-dense products, along with magazines touting the latest quickie diet. Fast-food restaurants tempt from nearly every street corner with takeout service—but nutrition is what they take out!

Many salads have as many calories as you get from one tablespoon of most salad dressings.

Modern food technology has turned inexpensive, low-calorie, high-volume foods into expensive, high-calorie, low-volume caloric bombs. It's now possible to eat a whole meal's worth of calories with only a few bites of food. No wonder people feel hungry and dissatisfied—and overeat!

How does it happen? Processing strips seven pounds of sugar beets of their bulk, fiber, and nutrients, producing one pound of pure sugar. Sugar and other refined sweeteners now account for more than 20 percent of daily calories eaten.

Technology takes 14 ears of corn and extracts one tablespoon of corn oil, which, along with its 110 calories, can be swallowed in one gulp! Extracted fats and oils account for another 20 percent of daily calories.

Grains, robbed of fiber and nutrients, can be turned into alcohol,

accounting for another 9 percent of empty calories many adults consume every day.

Add it up. About 50 percent of the modern Western diet consists of

Warning: Food processing may be hazardous to your health!

processed and concentrated calories devoid of vital nutrients and valuable fiber—a sure-fire formula for overweight.

So how do I go about losing weight?

If you love food but want to lose weight, then—

Eat more . . .
* Fresh and steamed vegetables,

but go easy on sauces and salad dressings.
* Whole grains—cooked cereals, brown rice, whole-grain breads and pasta.
  * Tubers and other vegetables—potatoes, yams, squash, and all kinds of beans, lentils, and peas.
  * Fresh, whole fruits.
    These foods "as grown" are filling, nutritious, inexpensive, and low in calories.

Eat less . . .
* Refined, processed, and concentrated foods. They are high in calories and price and low in nutrients and fiber.
* Nuts, meats, and rich dairy products. While these foods are nutritious, they have little fiber and bulk and are very high in fat and calories. Of the calories in meats and cheeses, for instance, 60 to 80 percent come from fat.

Anything else?
* *Drink plenty of water*—six to eight glasses a day. Try herb teas, mineral water, or just plain water. Keep the sodas for special occasions.
* *Walk briskly every day.* Keep at it until you can walk at least 30 minutes without fatigue or shortness of breath. Aim for 10,000 steps.
* *Beware of weak moments:*
  ~ If one cookie leads to a dozen, don't eat the first one.
  ~ Don't buy problem foods. If they are not around, you won't be tempted.
  ~ If you feel bored, frustrated,

or lonely, go for a walk, drink a glass of water, read a book, call a supportive friend. Or you can feast on natural foods, such as semifrozen grapes, juicy melons, or crunchy carrot sticks.

Fast-food restaurants tempt from nearly every street corner with takeout service—but what they take out is nutrition!

- *Tie in to spiritual resources.* God didn't make nobodies. He created you for health and prosperity.

It's time to put an end to those unbalanced semi-starvation diets that leave you frustrated, dissatisfied, and craving more to eat. Begin a lifestyle that will recondition your habits toward a lifetime of better health. By avoiding popular trends and choosing the right kinds of foods, you can eat more and still lose one to two pounds a week.

Extra pounds: Dietary Culprits

#1 Chips

They have contributed an estimated 8.5 lbs of extra weight in adults over the past 20 years.

#2 Soda Drinks

They have contributed an estimated 5 lbs of extra weight to adults over the same period.

NOTES

It is possible to eat as much as you want and still lose weight. The secret is knowing which foods to eat and which to avoid. Whole plant foods that promote good health and prevent disease are also ideal for taking weight off and keeping it off—for good.

Scared of a little broccoli?

Food Selection

For most of us, getting permanent control of a ballooning waistline requires a radical shift in diet. The table below summarizes the food selection principles presented in this book.

Weight Loss Tips: Attitude

Focus on the hundreds of foods that you can eat, not on those you shouldn't.

Be kind to yourself. It takes time to adapt to a new way of eating and living. Be patient and don't give up if you make a mistake or slip back into old habits. You are making a long-term investment in yourself. Keep going.

Your Challenge:

Begin to integrate everything you have found helpful in the past 10 lessons. You can release the slender person inside of you and enjoy a happier, healthier life.

Unit Review:

This is the last of 10 units devoted to weight control. As you have worked through them, we have encouraged you to try many new behaviors. Now that you have had a chance to experiment, we hope you will make them a permanent part of your life. (Take a look at the "Eight Steps" list to follow!.)

Eight Steps to Permanent Weight Control

1. Build your diet around fruits, vegetables, grains, legumes, and other "as grown" foods.

2. Forget "quickie" diets. Make the *Optimal Diet* your diet. *(See Coda, page 245.)*

3. Reduce the oils, butters, dressings and other fats you add to foods.

4. Read labels carefully and choose foods very low in fat, sugar, and salt.

5. Make water your drink of choice. Avoid high-calorie beverages.

6. Kick the snack habit. Begin each day with a hearty breakfast that makes midmorning snacking unnecessary.

7. Make exercise a part of your routine. Walk regularly. Aim for those 10,000 steps /day!

8. Develop a support network with others who share your interest in making positive lifestyle changes.

Eat freely from the following:

- **Fruit:** all fresh fruit (avocado and olives sparingly)
- **Vegetables:** all vegetables, greens, herbs, squash
- **Legumes:** all beans, peas, lentils, garbanzos
- **Tubers:** potatoes, yams, sweet potatoes
- **Whole Grains:** all grains, breads, pastas
- **Nuts:** use sparingly

"NOW THE Lord God had planted a garden in the east, in Eden; and there he put the [man and woman] he had formed. And the Lord God made all kinds of trees grow out of the ground—trees that were pleasing to the eye and good for food."–*Genesis 2:8, 9*

Natural Remedies

- **N**utrition
- **E**xercise
- **W**ater
- **S**unlight
- **T**emperance
- **A**ir
- **R**est
- **T**rust in Divine Power

The Ultimate Diet

Medicate yourself with food instead of pills.

Vegetarians are sprouting up all over—Over the last 15 years their number has tripled approaching now 19 million. As some 20 percent of Americans are now looking for restaurants with vegetarian menus. Once stereotyped as food fanatics or leftover hippies, vegetarians are now widely respected. They are considered healthier and their diet more ecologically sound.

Why go to the trouble of being a vegetarian?

Seven out of 10 Americans suffer and die prematurely of three killer diseases: heart disease, cancer, and stroke. Years ago, C. Everatt Koop, MD, then the US Surgeon General, unequivocally stated in his comprehensive report to the nation titled *Nutrition and Health*, that the rich Western diet was the major contributor to these diseases. He confirmed that saturated fat and cholesterol, eaten in disproportionate amounts, were the main culprits. He reminded people that animal products are the largest source of saturated fat as well as the only source of cholesterol. To compound the problem, Dr. Koop pointed out, these foods are usually eaten at the expense of unrefined complex-carbohydrate-rich foods, such as grains, legumes, and vegetables.

The average risk of heart disease for a man eating meat, eggs, and dairy products is 30 percent. The risk for a man who leaves off meat is 15 percent. However, the coronary risk of a vegetarian who leaves off meat, eggs, and dairy products drops to only 4 percent.

An editorial in the *Journal of the American Medical Association* commented on these advantages. It said, "A total vegetarian diet can prevent up to 90 percent of our strokes and 97 percent of our heart attacks."

Going beyond prevention, Dr. Dean Ornish, as well as Dr. Caldwell Esselstyn (from the cleveland Clinic) published studies proving, beyond a shadow of a doubt, that a very-low-fat vegetar-

> Seven out of 10 Americans suffer and die prematurely of three killer diseases; heart diesase, cancer, and stroke.

Breads and Cereals

These foods have a high complex-carbohydrate content and provide the body with energy. Sources: whole-grain bread, hot cereals, pasta, and brown rice.

Fruits and Veggies

This group is a primary source of phytochemicals and antioxidants, vitamins and minerals. Sources: for vitamin A, select dark-green, orange, or yellow vegetables; for vitamin C, select citrus fruits, strawberries, tomatoes, and potatoes.

Legumes

Beans rate high in soluble fiber, protein, and energy, as well as phytochemicals and anti-oxidants. Because they contain a plant hormone called phytoestrogens, soybeans are hard to beat among the beans.

ian diet could *reverse* heart disease in patients scheduled for coronary bypass surgery.

The risk for cancer of the prostate, breast, and colon is three to four times higher for people who consume meat, eggs, and dairy products on a daily basis when compared to those who eat them sparingly or not at all. In addition, vegetarian women have stronger bones and fewer fractures, and they lose less bone as they age.

Studies of long-lived vegetarian people, healthy and active into advanced age, contrast sharply with the short life spans and increased disease rates of traditional Eskimos, who depend largely on what they catch from the sea.

Are there significant ecological effects?

Shifting toward a vegetarian lifestyle would greatly ease the environmental impact of our present meat-centered diet. According to a recent United Nations report, pollution from animal-based agriculture is greater than from all other human and industrial activities combined. Overgrazing and intense cultivation of land for production of animal foods contributes substantially to the massive erosion and the irretrievable loss of 6 billion tons of valuable topsoil annually in America.

But the impact of a meat-centered diet goes beyond North America. In the 1970s, in Central America, for example, irreparable damage with global implications took place on a daily basis. Americans then ate more than 200 million pounds of Central American beef every year. Powerful landowners destroyed nearly half the region's rain forests, turning them into grazing lands for the cattle

The Dallas . . . Vegeboys?

A few years ago the Super Bowl-winning Dallas Cowboys were rated the healthiest team in the NFL by the Professional Football Athletic Trainers Society. How did they do it? The players ate six daily servings of fruits and vegetables along with plenty of low-fat, grain-based foods such as bread and spaghetti.

Gone are the seasons during which beefy linebackers thought they had to eat a steady diet of red meat.

The National Cancer Institute Recommends Nine a Day

To tap the healing power of fruits and vegetables, you have to help yourself to enough servings. Most Americans don't. Do you?

Did you eat your fruits and vegetables today?

needed to supply the ever-expanding hamburger chains. It took 55 square feet of land to produce a single pound of hamburger. And the tragic story repeats itself today in Brazil, where half of the Amazon Rain Forest — the "green lungs" of planet Earth — is being taken out to create grazing land for cattle!

Doesn't this impact the world's food supplies?

By moving away from a meat-centered diet, we could use our grains and beans to feed the world's hungry people instead of the world's cattle and poultry. The amount of land needed to feed one person consuming a meat-based diet would feed 20 vegetarians. One acre of land yields only 183 pounds of beef, but 20,000 pounds of potatoes. To produce one pound of edible flesh from a feedlot steer requires 10 pounds of grain and soybeans. It's a poor conversion system that operates at a 10 percent efficiency level!

Are vegetarians able to meet their nutrient needs?

Easily. The Recommended Daily Intake (RDI) for protein is 45 to 60 grams for adults, which works out to about 10

to 12 percent of calories eaten. A beefsteak offers about 25 percent of its calories as usable protein. The protein content of grains usually exceeds 10 percent of total calories, and dried beans and peas actually carry close to 25 percent of their calories as usable protein. Even vegetables average about 20 percent of their calories as protein. So there is plenty of protein in plant foods, which are also low in fat, high in fiber, and cholesterol-free.

Studies show that complementary proteins, iron and calcium supplies are essentially nonproblems in humans eating a variety of plant foods, although pure vegetarians may require small supplements of vitamin B_{12}.

Will switching to a vegetarian diet affect my weight?

If you replace the meat in your diet with doughnuts, Twinkies, french fries, and other high-fat, high-sugar morsels, then, yes, you will probably gain weight.

If you choose, however, to eat more foods-as-grown, simply prepared, without those nutrition-depleted calories, you can shed excess weight and stabilize at a healthier level.

Any suggestions for making the transition?

Some people can switch to a vegetarian diet cold turkey, but others do it more gradually, eliminating red meat first, then poultry, fish, and finally dairy products.

Another idea is to begin with one or more meatless days a week. As you experiment with vegetarian dishes, you can gradually increase the number of meatless meals.

Switching to a less meat-centered diet is really not such a big deal. We already eat bean burritos, pasta, and other standard meatless fare. Stretch your imagination. Enjoy the varied tastes. Save on your food dollar. And savor a new level of health.

The evidence against meat continues to grow as it once did for cigarettes. The plant food-centered diet is proving to be the ultimate diet—maximizing health, preventing disease, releasing food to the hungry, and preserving the planet. It's increasingly being viewed as being smart, healthy, caring, economically sound — and it is considered to be a responsible choice! Isn't it time for Americans to stop slaughtering 1 million creatures every hour for food?

Application

Vegetarians are no longer viewed as food fanatics and counterculture oddballs. Studies confirm that most live longer, healthier lives, and they leave a softer footprint on the earth—they are ecologically tuned in. Making the transition to a meat-free diet can be a challenging adventure, leading to a new level of good health and well-being.

The Optimal Diet

By now you have been exposed to the *Optimal Diet* several times. Here are some questions to see how much you remember:

1. Are animal products necessary for good health and nutrition?
   __ Yes
   __ No

2. What is the average risk of heart disease for a man eating meat, eggs, and dairy products?
   __ 15 percent
   __ 30 percent
   __ 45 percent
   __ 75 percent

3. On average, vegetarians are:
   __ Heavier than meat eaters
   __ Thinner than meat eaters
   __ Weigh the same as meat eaters

4. Where do most of the calories in meat come from?
   __ Fat
   __ Protein
   __ Carbohydrates

5. Where is cholesterol found?
   __ All foods
   __ Peanut butter
   __ All animal products
   __ Plant foods

6. Meat-centered diets have been linked with:
   __ Heart disease
   __ Stroke
   __ Cancer
   __ All of the above

Lunch on the Go

For busy people, lunch is often a difficult meal. The temptation is to grab something quick. Fortunately, quick does not have to mean a burger from a fast-food restaurant. With some advance planning, you can take a healthful lunch wherever you go.

Your Challenge:

Meat can be hazardous to your health. Start eliminating it from your diet by making your own delicious lunches.

1. No **2.** 30 percent **3.** Thinner than meat eaters **4.** Fat **5.** All animal products **6.** All of the above

NOTES

_____

_____

_____

_____

_____

_____

Modern Fountain of Youth

A healthful lifestyle can hold back the aging processes as much as 30 years.

T he fabled fountain of youth lured ancient adventurers into a lifetime of fruitless searching. In time it became a symbol for an impossible dream. That was yesterday. Today science seems able to put at least part of this dream within reach of nearly all of us.

What do you mean?

When the explorers were searching for a secret spring that would maintain perpetual youth, many people were dying in early adulthood of infectious diseases. Today improved sanitation and hygiene, along with antibiotics and vaccines, have almost eliminated those diseases. The battle has now shifted to lifestyle diseases. These are the maladies that are now robbing us of our energy, disabling us prematurely, and killing us s-l-o-w-l-y.

The good news is that greater vitality, better health, and longer life can be ours through regular, brisk physical activity.

Do you mean EXERCISE? Can it really do all that?

Take a look at the facts. The adage "Use it or lose it" applies not only to muscles and bones but also to hearts, lungs, brains, blood vessels, joints, and every other part of the body. A sedentary lifestyle is a direct route to an earlier grave. Inactivity kills us—literally.

Just being thin and "hip" isn't enough anymore. To be beautiful today, you have to be healthy and fit. And to be healthy and fit, you've got to exercise.

A strong genetic inheritance helps some people survive incredible odds. But just living longer isn't today's only concern. Along with their lengthened years people are looking for energy, good health, usefulness, and quality of life.

> **"The Lord God took the man and put him in the Garden of Eden to work it and take care of it."**
> —Genesis 2:15

Just how does physical exercise help us live longer and better?

Here are some of the ways:

- Exercise helps us FEEL GOOD! Life becomes more fun, and the high that comes from exercise won't let you down later. Moreover, the hormones producing the exercise high are proving to be health-promoting as well.
- Exercise strengthens the heart. This is important in a culture in which every second person dies of heart and vascular disease.
- Exercise lowers blood pressure and resting heart rate, protecting the heart and blood vessels.
- Exercise lowers LDL cholesterol levels in the blood and often raises HDL cholesterol, again decreasing heart and vascular risk. (LDL is the bad part of cholesterol; HDL is the good part.)
- Exercise strengthens bones by helping retain calcium and other minerals.
- Exercise lifts depression. Outdoor exercise is one of the most valu-

able tools for fighting this common and disabling malady.

- Exercise relieves anxiety and stress. In our harried, pressured society, physical activity is proving to be an effective antidote.
- Exercise increases overall

In today's world, sweat is status and trimness is success. More and more modern executives are apt to be in prime condition.

energy and efficiency in all areas of our lives.

- Exercise helps maintain desirable weight levels. It builds muscles and burns fat. Moderate exercise blunts appetite by temporarily increasing blood sugar levels.
- Exercise improves circulation, and that makes for clearer minds, better sleep, and faster healing of damaged body areas.

What kind of exercise are you talking about? Not everyone can jog, or run marathons.

Every one of these listed benefits can come from plain, simple walking. Walking is the ideal exercise. It's inexpensive. It's safe. Nearly everyone can do it. And it's fun! You can select your own speed, and you can stop when you want. As your fitness improves, you can gradually add speed and time.

Other good exercises are swimming, bicycling, gardening, yard work, and golf—if you leave the carts behind. For hardier souls, jogging, stair climbing, rock climbing, jumping rope, and skiing provide challenging variations. In bad weather, try stationary bicycles, trampolines, rowing machines, or simply walking or jogging in place. To be effective, active (aerobic) exercise should be brisk and continuous for at least 15 to 20 minutes. Most people can work up to this goal. A daily program of 30 to 40 minutes of active exercise will give you maximum benefits. To lose weight, and for diabetics needing to control their blood sugar, increase the time to one hour. You can divide the hour into two or three sessions if you wish.

Is it true that reaching a certain pulse rate is necessary for exercise to be effective?

There are exercise regimes for specific purposes. The concept of training heart rate is particularly useful in strengthening the heart. Weight and flexibility training is also

HOPE FOR THE COUCH POTATO

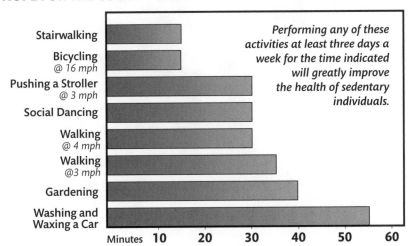

Performing any of these activities at least three days a week for the time indicated will greatly improve the health of sedentary individuals.

Health Note

Women who log at least four hours of exercise a week cut their risk of breast cancer by more than a third. Active people are about half as liable to get colon cancer as are inactive people.

Put more zest in your life!

proving to be valuable. Remember: even moderate activities, such as brisk walking, will improve fitness. Every step counts. And health-promoting agencies recommend 10,000 steps/day.

But I hate to exercise. It's boring!

We all do many boring things every day: brushing our teeth, cleaning the house, washing the car, mowing the lawn, doing dishes, going to work. But we do these things because we like the rewards: beautiful teeth, an attractive home, a clean car, a regular paycheck. After a while these activities become routine, an accepted part of our daily living.

Let's look at exercise the same way. Its benefits are far greater than a clean house—they last a lifetime.

Easy Ways to Stay Fit for Life

Exercise slows down the aging process. It strengthens the heart, lowers blood pressure, relieves stress, preserves muscle function, and helps you maintain a desirable weight. You don't need expensive equipment or a health club membership to start. Walking can provide all these benefits and more.

The 10-Step Exercise Program

Have you tried exercise before and found that you just couldn't stick with it? If so, you should try the world's easiest exercise system. It's called the 10-Step Program.

All you do is make a commitment to the first 10 steps of a daily walk. That's it. You get out and take those steps every day. Once they're behind you, you can turn around and go home, if you wish.

The system works because it eases you past those difficult first steps. It gets you up and going. And if you are like most people, once you get going you will finish the entire walk.

The 10-Step Program also keeps you in the habit of exercising even when you can't manage your full routine. You might be sick, or traveling, yet in almost every situation you can manage 10 steps. In this way you maintain the exercise habit even when you can't exercise. That's important if you want to enjoy the benefits of fitness for the rest of your life.

Plan Ahead

A useful technique is to plan your exercise sessions in advance. If you are an early riser, try exercising be-fore breakfast. If your morning is already too full, walk during your lunch hour or in the evening. The important thing is to find a time that is right for you.

People Make Exercise Fun

Many people complain that exercise is boring. To liven up your sessions, include friends and family members in your exercise activities. If they won't join you, take the dog out for a stroll. Exercise can be enjoyable if you approach it with an attitude of fun and creativity.

Your Challenge:

Schedule your exercise sessions in advance and use the 10-Step Program to get you moving. Regular exercise is as necessary as air, water, and wholesome food. Don't let another day go by without it.

A newer concept for fitness recommends:

- Aerobic exercise for 30 minutes three times weekly.

- Alternate with 30 minutes of strength and flexibility training three times a week.

NOTES

The No-Calorie Wonder

Forcing the body to work with limited amounts of fluid is like trying to wash the dinner dishes in a cupful of water. When you don't drink enough water, the body must excrete wastes in a much more concentrated form, causing body odor, bad breath, and unpleasant-smelling urine.

Don't most people get the water they need?

It's been said that the French don't drink water, only wine. We smile at this, but it's becoming a reality in America today. Our kids are drowning in soft drinks—soda pop has become their main beverage. The average teenager downs two to three cans a day, and some as many as six and seven. Many adults drink more beer than water. In addition, plenty of tea, coffee, and other beverages are consumed.

Notice what happens next time you go to a restaurant for a meal. You will usually be served a glass of ice water and then asked expectantly, "And what would you like to drink?"

How many glasses of just plain water does the average American drink? The truth for many is—hardly any.

Does it matter what beverages I drink? They all contain water, don't they?

Our bodies are about 70 percent water, and our kidneys process more than 47 gallons of it in a day. Without it we'd look more wrinkled than a California prune!

But why is this colorless, tasteless, calorie-and-salt-free substance so absolutely necessary?

The answer lies in the physiological workings of the body. Water to the body is like oil to a car engine. It's the magic lubricant that makes

> Our bodies are about 70 percent water, and our kidneys process more than 47 gallons of it in a day.

everything else work. A drink of water is exactly what the body needs to carry out all its life processes.

Beverages other than water, however, pose special problems. Many have calories that must be digested like food. Such calories may produce extra fat, blood sugar swings, and a slowed digestion. Many beverages increase the secretion of acid in the stomach. Some popular sodas contain phosphoric acid that can help deplete the body's calcium supplies, thus contributing to brittle bones.

Sugar in beverages requires extra water for metabolism. Recent studies have demonstrated that caffeine and alcohol dehydrate the body because they work as diuretics. This can contribute to fatigue, dry skin, indigestion, and headaches. The solution? For every alcoholic drink, for every cup of coffee, for every cola, be sure you drink an extra glass of water.

Do the "no sugar" diet drinks solve these problems?

Diet beverages don't contain sugar, but they present other concerns. Nearly all beverages, sugared or not, contain chemicals that are added for color, flavor, preservation, and other reasons. Some of these may irritate delicate stomach linings, and some may also require the liver and kidneys to detoxify and dispose of them.

Drinking water eliminates all of these problems. It has no extra calories to slow down digestion or to add unwanted fat. It has no irritants to stress the sensitive linings of the digestive tract, fewer chemicals to threaten delicate body machinery, and no caffeine. It's readily available, and it's cheap!

How much water should I drink?

Drink enough to keep the urine pale. The body loses about 10 to 12 cups of water a day through the skin, lungs, urine, and feces. Food provides two to four cups of water, leaving us about eight glasses of water to drink.

Get into the habit of drinking water liberally. Drink on arising, and in midmorning and midafternoon. A drink of water is like an internal shower. It rinses the stomach and prepares it for its work.

DO YOU WANT CAFFEINE?
(per 12-ounce serving)

Monster Drink	120 mg
Java Water	100 mg
Jolt	100 mg
Mountain Dew	54 mg
Coca-Cola	45 mg
Pepsi-Cola	40 mg

So start the day right. Give that early-morning drink some zest by adding a twist of lemon. Then during morning and afternoon coffee breaks, reach for a glass of water and drink to your body's content. Tempted to snack? Replace it with a drink of water. It's magic!

Water is the perfect beverage, and one of life's greatest blessings. The next time you are asked, "Anything to drink?" you can say, "Yes, a glass of water is fine. In fact, it's perfect."

Bottled? or Tap?

With reports of contamination by heavy metals, nuclear wastes, fertilizers, pesticides, herbicides, and leak-

Some Alternatives to Tap Water

Bulk waters sold in one-gallon jugs are the most popular. These are often processed from ordinary tap water. If you want water from protected springs and wells, look for words such as "spring," "artesian," or "mineral water" on the label.

Mineral waters contain dissolved minerals, sometimes natural, sometimes added.

Sparkling water is a generic term for any carbonated water. Some, like club sodas, are relatively high in sodium and should not be used by people with high blood pressure.

Seltzer water refers to filtered, carbonated tap water that has no added mineral salts. Many, however, have added sugars, up to 100 calories per eight ounces.

Distilled water is the purest. All minerals have been removed, either by distillation or by osmosis, leaving the water tasting rather flat. It's the hardness of the water—the minerals—that gives water its flavor.

Heartburn?

Drink some water every half hour. This will give you a regular stress break, and it will also wash the acid out of your esophagus and dilute it.

ing fuels—some people are afraid to drink the water that comes out of their kitchen faucet.

With good reason, wouldn't you say?

Many Americans think so. Consumers spent $5.2 billion last year on bottled waters. But are they getting what they are paying for?

One problem is that the federal and state requirements are exactly the same for both bottled and tap water. Another concern is the absence of fluoride in bottled watter. Also, once opened, bottled water may be more vulnerable to bacteria because of the absence of chlorine.

Since most municipal systems are tested daily, if your water supply is up to standard, what comes out of your faucet may be just as safe as the bottled water you buy. And it's hundreds of times cheaper!

What can I do if my tap water is unsafe?

One way you can protect yourself is by installing your own filtering system: a good charcoal filter removes most contaminants and makes the water taste good.

If you depend on private wells, your local government may test your water for a nominal fee. National mail-order testing services are also available.

But bottled waters taste so much better!

Sometimes they do, but not always. If you are willing to pay, there are many alternative choices (see sidebar on page 191).

The irony of it all is that most of us face more health hazards from not drinking enough water than we do from its possible contaminants.

NOTES

Today North Americans drink more soft drinks and alcoholic beverages than water. These substitutes force the body to deal with calories and chemicals, and can disturb the process of digestion. The body needs water to function properly. When you want refreshment, choose the real thing—water.

Most People Should Drink More

Water really is the most healthful drink. We can live only a few days in its absence. Even though we all get enough to sustain us, most people don't drink enough for optimum functioning. We sip enough to survive, when we should be drinking enough to thrive. The result is unnecessary stress placed on the body's cleansing system and other functions.

Start Early

One way to make sure you get your daily quota is by drinking two glasses of water when you wake up in the morning. Do this before you get caught up in the activities of the day. With two glasses down, you need to drink only six more during the rest of the day. That is a feat everyone can manage. If you wait until you are thirsty, you probably won't get enough.

Worried About Contaminants?

In most cases the health hazards we face from not drinking enough water are greater than those from possible contaminants in the water supply. If you are concerned, have your water tested, or install a good charcoal filter. A filter helps purify your water and makes it taste better.

Fighting Where the Battle Is

What makes more sense, eating fruits and vegetables needed for good health, or avoiding them on the off chance that they may contain pesticide residue?

Likewise, what makes more sense, drinking the eight glasses of water that your body needs to flush out toxins, or avoiding tap water for fear that it may contain something dangerous? Be good to yourself: start enjoying nature's super fluid today.

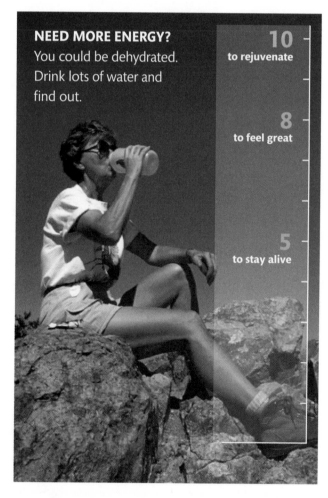

NEED MORE ENERGY?
You could be dehydrated. Drink lots of water and find out.

10
to rejuvenate

8
to feel great

5
to stay alive

NOTES

Kiss of the Sun

Excessive exposure to sunlight can cause skin cancer as well as premature wrinkling and aging of the skin. In proper amounts, however, the sun's rays can be good for your health.

You say "proper amounts." Can sunlight be measured?

Yes. It's important to understand the power of sunlight. Most of us have observed how dim even the brightest electric lightbulb appears in daylight. The intensity of light is measured in "lux," or "luxes." For example, outdoor light can reach 3,000 lux on a bright sunny day. A bright indoor environment may provide only 400 lux, less than 15 percent of daylight brightness.

In recent years melatonin, a natural body hormone, has been found to enhance sleep. Melatonin levels reach a peak in children, and fall slowly and steadily throughout adult life. This may explain why children sleep so much better than older people.

The body carefully regulates melatonin production. The process is largely controlled by the light-dark cycle. Optimal melatonin production occurs only at night, in a dark environment. The pineal gland, located in the center of the brain, is the "clock" that regulates this process at the right time.

Melatonin is not stored in the body. We need a liberal supply each evening to sleep well. Studies demonstrate that daily exposure to natural sunlight will boost melatonin output. Artificial light is a weak substitute, as are manufactured supplements.

Besides improving sleep, what else does sunlight have to offer?

Sunlight is an efficient germ killer. That's why it is important to sun and air out blankets, quilts, and other items that are not washed regularly and sterilized in an automatic dryer.

Proper amounts of sunshine also give the skin a healthy glow and

Sunlight elevates the mood for most people, producing a sense of well-being. Combined with active exercise, sunshine is an important adjunct in treating acute and chronic depressions.

help make it smooth and pliable. A moderately tanned skin is more resistant to infections and sunburns than untanned skin.

Also, sunlight elevates the mood for most people, producing a sense of well-being. (Just don't stay out too long and get sunburned!) Combined with active exercise, sunshine is an important adjunct in treating acute and chronic depressions. Remember, when depressed during winter's cold and gloomy months, try to catch any possible ray of sunshine.

What's more, the body is able to manufacture vitamin D by the action of sunlight on the skin. It's called the "sunshine vitamin"—just 15 minutes of sun exposure to your face and arms will provide a jolt of 20,000 Int. Units (IU) of Vitamin D. That's much more than the recommended 600 IU to be taken in by diet. Vitamin D enables the body to pick up calcium from the intestines for use in building healthy bones. It prevents both childhood and adult rickets and aids in the prevention of osteoporosis.

Sunlight also helps to:
- enhance the immune system
- alleviate pain from swollen arthritic joints
- relieve certain symptoms of PMS

Most of us no longer wake up with the dawn, spend the day outdoors, and sleep when it's dark.

- lower blood cholesterol levels

Is there a flip side?

Sunlight is a major risk factor for skin cancer, especially in light-skinned people. Too much sunlight, for them may be particularly damaging.

You should also know that burning the skin is extremely harmful for everyone. Every burn destroys healthy living tissue. Repeated burns cause irreversible damage and can set up a person for skin cancer.

And if all that isn't bad enough, repeated sunburn and even repeated

deep tanning of the skin gradually destroy its elasticity and its oil glands, producing wrinkling and premature aging.

Some studies suggest that a high-fat diet, when combined with exposure to sunlight, may also promote cancers of the skin.

What are some guidelines for safe, healthy exposure to sunlight?
- Modest tanning is protective, like putting sunglasses on your skin. But you must understand your own tolerance to sunlight. Fair-skinned people and redheads may have to begin with only five minutes of exposure to the sun per day. Darker-skinned people can begin with 10 to 15 minutes per day. Up to 30 minutes of sunshine, exposing as much of the body as possible, is a realistic goal for most people.
- Never, never burn! Malignant melanoma, the deadliest form of skin cancer, kills nearly 7,000

Did You Know?

- An extra hour of light a day may lift your spirits and affect your energy, sleep, fertility, and even PMS.

- Seasonal variations in light levels can have a profound effect on mental health. This is clearest in people suffering from seasonal affective disorder (SAD)—a depressive illness that is successfully treated with light therapy.

- People getting more sunshine are less likely to get breast, colon, or prostate cancer.

Earth is a solar-powered world, 98 percent of its warmth coming from sunshine (the rest from geothermal heat). Solar energy lifts rain clouds, drives winds, and sparks the photosynthesis in plants, which feed all living things.

For thousands of years sunlight has been known as a mediator of life. But we know today that it can be healing or destructive; it can be the kiss of life or the kiss of death, depending on how we use it.

NASA uses bright light exposure to reset biological rhythms of the astronauts to decrease rocket lag (and jet lag).

Americans a year; squamous cell carcinoma, more than 2,000. Sunburns raise the risk of both. A study in Israel found that Orthodox Jews, who wear coats and hats or shawls year-round, were much less prone to melanoma than were Israelis who regularly exposed their skin to the sun.

Wear protective clothing, eyewear, and a protective sunscreen if needed. Be especially careful around snow or water and on cloudy days.

- If you have an outdoor trip or vacation coming up, prepare your skin by giving it progressive exposure in the days beforehand, to the point of pinking up.
- A few minutes of sunshine on your face and hands each day will produce all the vitamin D you need.
- Open up your house to the sunshine each morning. It will improve your health and lift your spirits.
- Just remember that artificial light is a very poor substitute for the real thing. Where possible, spend a little time each day soaking up some daylight.

NOTES

Application

Sunshine can be good for you. It kills germs, helps improve your mood, and allows the body to produce vitamin D. Yet while some exposure is good, too much can destroy the skin's elasticity and increase the risk of skin cancer. Enjoy sunlight and outside activities, but protect yourself from overexposure.

Friend or Foe?

Over the past few years, articles about the effects of the sun and the danger of skin cancer have driven many people into the dark. That's not all bad. Certainly you should use caution to avoid burning, but to avoid the sun altogether deprives you of one of nature's great healing remedies.

It's good to spend at least a few minutes in the sunshine every day. Studies have shown that for some people, lack of exposure to light causes depression. Taking a sunshine break will give your body a dose of vitamin D and will act as a disinfectant, killing bacteria on your clothes and skin.

During the summer do you:
__ sizzle and sunburn?
__ work on a deep, dark tan?
__ tan lightly?
__ stay out of the sun completely?

If you sizzle and burn or go for that deep tan, watch out! You are putting yourself at risk for skin cancer and damaging the elasticity of your skin.

On the other hand, lightly tanned skin is more resistant to sunburn and less prone to infection. Get outside in the fresh air. Soak up a little sunshine each day; just don't overdo it.

Ask Yourself

How often do you spend time in the sunshine?
__ every day, weather permitting
__ most days
__ a few times a week
__ rarely

Sunlight Suggestions

1. Avoid going to sleep in the sun. It's a recipe for a severe sunburn.

2. Use sunscreen and sunglasses to protect yourself. A hat is also helpful to shade your face when you are working outdoors.

3. Be extra careful when you are around water or snow. The reflection from these surfaces can increase your exposure, causing you to burn rapidly.

4. If you are swimming, remember to reapply your sunscreen when you are done. Better yet, use waterproof sunscreen.

Open up your windows and let the sunshine in.

It will kill germs, lift your spirits, and enhance your health.

NOTES

The Balanced Life

It was headline news: Carrots may prevent head and neck cancer. New research suggested that eating five or six of the crunchy tubers a day appeared to reverse leukoplakia—a precancerous lesion occurring in the mouth and throat.

My friend Judith promptly purchased a machine that turned fresh carrots into juice.

"How much juice do you get from five carrots?" I asked her one day.

Her eyes flashed. "Oh, I don't stop there. With this machine I can drink five or six pounds of carrots every day!"

Was that a good idea?

It's true that vegetables are an important part of a healthful diet. It's also true that they are increasingly being valued for their role in preventing disease.

But five pounds of one vegetable every day?

Judith's body eventually rebelled. Her skin took on a sickly yellowish color. Fearing hepatitis, she rushed to the doctor. He explained that carrots contain an orange-yellow dye known as beta-carotene. The body handles reasonable quantities of this substance, but excessive amounts are stashed away in the liver, skin, and muscous membranes, turning them the color of a carrot.

Did that experience straighten her out?

For the moment. But we humans are a curious lot. Sensationalized discoveries and quick solutions to complex health problems are almost irresistible. Before the carrot caper, Judith was swept into the excitement over oat bran. After months of mush and muffins, however, she was ready for a change.

> People do nearly everything to excess—they eat too much, drink too much, smoke too much, spend too much, party too much. Moderation is about as popular a concept as wholesome.

Do carrots actually protect us from cancer?

Carrots and other yellow fruits and vegetables are rich in beta-carotene, the substance that began to change Judith's skin color. Beta-carotene, which the body turns into vitamin A, is also a substance that appears to protect the body against certain cancers.

Vitamins can be divided into two basic types—those that are water-soluble (dissolve in water) and those that are fat-soluble (dissolve in fat). Water-soluble vitamins (B-complex and C) are not a special concern, because excess amounts can usually be washed out through the kidneys.

But fat-soluble vitamins (A, D, E, and K) are another story. Any excess cannot be eliminated except as it is used. In excessive amounts, vitamin A begins to act like a toxin (poison) and may cause headaches, joint pains, damaged skin, and hair loss.

Because of this potential toxicity, laws now limit the amount of vitamin A and other fat-soluble vitamins that can be put into supplements.

> In a survey of Americans over age 90, 95 percent said that they don't smoke, and 88 percent reported that they don't drink.

Beta-carotene apparently doesn't have such limits. When the body receives beta-carotene it can make as much vitamin A as it needs and use the rest in other ways. That's why the trend these days is to substitute beta-carotene for vitamin A in vitamin capsules and tablets.

This distinction is important because it illustrates how the body uses food. Vitamins, minerals, and other nutrients in natural food occur in exactly the right forms for the body to use. It can pick and choose what it needs. But when we consume one food or nutrient in excess, or tamper with the makeup of food, the whole balance can be upset.

So beta-carotene is good, but a whole lot of it isn't necessarily better.

This is a hard message for today's world. People do nearly everything to excess—they eat too much, drink too much, smoke too much, spend too much, party too much. Moderation is about as popular a concept as wholesome.

Then too, we live in an instant society with a quick-fix mentality, and it's difficult to accept that instant good health isn't also available. Each

The Key Is Balance

"I have never seen a person who died of old age. In fact, I do not think anyone has ever died of old age yet. To die of old age would mean that all the organs of the body had worn out proportionally, merely by having been used too long. This is never the case. We invariably die because one vital part has worn out too early in proportion to the rest of the body.

"There is always one part that wears out first and wrecks the whole human machinery, merely because the other parts cannot function without it.

"The lesson seems to be that as far as man can regulate his life by voluntary actions, he should seek to equalize stress throughout his being.

"The human body—like the tires on a car or the rug on a floor—wears longest when it wears evenly."

—*Dr. Hans Selye*

> **A balanced, healthful lifestyle may not grab headlines or create profitable markets, but it brings improved health that lasts.**

time a new fad splashes through the media there's no shortage of takers.

As consultants for a health publication, we get a lot of phone calls from reporters. They often try to get us to say such things as "Yes, eating a pound of alfalfa sprouts every day will strengthen the heart" or "Several capsules of rooted seaweed will ensure a good night's sleep." No one wants to hear our message about the good-sense, balanced diet the body really needs. We soon realized that even though we were giving them the right stuff, a healthful, balanced lifestyle didn't grab headlines, sell magazines (even health magazines), or create profitable new markets for food products.

The human body is able to tolerate excesses of one kind or another for a long time—even six pounds of carrots a day! But the bottom line is that balance, not only in what we eat, but in our total lifestyle, is the key to enduring health and happiness.

NOTES

Application

Too much of a good thing is a bad thing when your health is involved. Common sense and moderation will do more for you than any health fad or miracle cure. Balance is the key to good health—learn to apply it in all areas of your life.

The Case of the Harried Sales Manager

Joe is a sales manager for a telecommunications company. At work he is always busy, talking with customers, motivating his sales team, or writing reports for a demanding boss. The pressure never lets up. For lunch he has a steak and salad if there are clients to entertain, or else he grabs a double cheeseburger and fries at a nearby fast-food restaurant. Sometimes there's no time for lunch at all. By the time Joe gets home at night, he's exhausted and cranky. "I feel like a wreck," he admits. "After work, all I want is to relax in front of the television. I know I should make some changes, but I'm not sure how to start."

Balance Is "Common Sense in Action"

Imagine that Joe came to you for advice. What commonsense changes might you suggest to help him incorporate the principle of balance in his life?

_____

_____

_____

_____

Joe's Solution

Joe made a couple simple changes in his routine. First, he started bringing his lunch to work instead of eating out every day. Packing a lunch made it easy to eat more fruits, vegetables, and whole-grain foods, and helped him cut down on high-fat, high-calorie, restaurant fare. Second, Joe and his wife, Amy, now take a brisk walk in the evening when he gets home.

When asked if the changes have been worth it, Joe smiles. "I feel more relaxed and energetic. I've lost weight, and the walks Amy and I take together have become something we both look forward to. It's hard to believe the dramatic impact these changes have made in my life."

How About You?

What are some things you could do starting today to bring more balance to this part of your life? List your ideas:

_____

_____

_____

NOTES

_____

_____

_____

_____

_____

_____

Don't Poison Your Home

H ouseplants do a lot more than enhance the appearance of our homes and offices. They enrich the air with oxygen and absorb carbon dioxide; some even remove toxic pollutants from the air we breathe.

You mean harmful pollutants can collect indoors?

Increasingly so. Many modern homes and office buildings are tightly sealed to save energy costs. But this advantage may be offset by poor ventilation and potential accumulation of indoor air pollutants.

Tobacco smoke, of course, is the most dangerous pollutant, but there are others.

Formaldehyde, for example, seeps from certain wood products, and other chemical fumes come from carpeting, copy machines, upholstery, cleaning products, and freshly dry-cleaned clothes. Carbon monoxide and nitrogen dioxide, two poisonous gases, may come from gas, oil, and coal furnaces, gas ranges, fireplaces, and kerosene heaters.

Other problems occur from dust, air mites, molds and fungi, ozone, lead, asbestos, pesticide residues, and, in some areas, radon gas.

How do these pollutants affect people?

Symptoms range from burning eyes, sore throats, coughing, and itching, to headaches, sluggishness, nausea, dizziness, feelings of exhaustion, and depression. This cluster of symptoms is sometimes referred to as "sick building syndrome."

Air conveys life, vigor, and electrifying energy to every cell in the body.

A "feel good" technique is to stop where you are and take a few slow, deep breaths several times a day. This gives your body and extra "shot of oxygen" and helps unload carbon dioxide.

What can people do to protect themselves?

There are two basic ways to protect ourselves, not 100 percent, but significantly.

First, we can control exposure. For example:

- Ban smoking indoors. Even secondhand smoke contains hundreds of harmful chemicals.
- Make sure all gas, oil, kerosene, and coal-burning heaters and appliances, as well as coal- and wood-burning furnaces and fireplaces, are properly vented to the outdoors. And don't forget gas cooking ranges and clothes dryers.
- Keep heating and air-conditioning units well maintained. Clean air ducts and filters regularly.
- Keep chimneys open and in good repair.
- Use air fresheners, moth crystals, etc., sparingly.
- Avoid idling a vehicle in an attached garage or near an open window.

Second, we can improve ventilation.

The most obvious solution to indoor pollution problems is to open windows and set up good cross ventilation. Fresh air not only dilutes trapped fumes, thus decreasing their health threats, but enriches stale air as well. People often don't realize that in closed areas the same air can be breathed and rebreathed, over and

Are you getting enough vitamin O_2?

over. The oxygen content decreases, and the carbon dioxide and other wastes increase, resulting in sleepiness, sluggishness, and headaches.

Here are some suggestions:

- Set air conditioners and heating systems to bring in 20 to 35 percent (or more) fresh air. Energy costs will be somewhat higher, but health benefits will more than compensate for this.
- Air out your house at least once a day. On smoggy days, air out the house at night or in the early mornings. In most areas smog particulate matter drops considerably once the sun has set.
- Sleep with an open window. Set up cross ventilation in your bedroom if possible. You'll wake up feeling refreshed.

What about air-cleaning machines?

These machines can be expensive, complicated, and messy, and most have a limited range. However, people with allergies and certain lung ailments often find them helpful. And we recommend them for anyone exposed to air polluted with tobacco smoke at home or at work.

How does air relate to personal health?

Air is composed of about 20 percent oxygen, the rest being nitrogen, along with a few other gases. Since the human body operates on oxygen, each one of its 100 trillion cells must receive steady, fresh supplies, or die. Oxygen is picked up in the lungs from the air we breathe, and delivered to our bodies via the red blood cells. Well-oxygenated cells are healthy and contribute to overall well-being. Anything that diminishes oxygen supplies to the lungs, or its delivery to body cells, is detrimental.

Air molecules can also be positively or negatively charged. Polluted air is usually full of positive ions. It's commonly found on freeways, at airports, and in closed, poorly ventilated areas.

Air Is the Breath of Life

We are fully dependent on it for oxygen to operate the powerhouses in our cells. These powerhouses, called mitochondria, are the backbone of every activity carried on in our bodies.

The heart sends blood streaming on its way, filled with red blood cells whose hemoglobin picks up fresh oxygen in the lungs and delivers it to every cell in the body.

Oxygen is vital to each of the trillions of cells that make up your body. Poor breathing habits, or poor air to breathe, can rob the body of this vital element. Bad air and poor breathing habits promote negative emotions, such as depression and irritability. It can also cause headaches and chronic feelings of fatigue and exhaustion.

Air containing an abundance of negative ions is plentiful around lakes, in forests, near rivers and waterfalls, at the seashore, and after a rainstorm. This kind of air is refreshing and gives people a lift.

Another "feel good" technique is to stop where you are and take a few slow, deep breaths several times a day. This gives your body an extra "shot of oxygen" and helps unload carbon dioxide.

Yet another way to flush your body with oxygen is to exercise. Activity opens up blood vessels and speeds those oxygen-laden red blood cells on their rounds.

And remember the houseplants. Placing at least one plant for every 100 square feet of indoor space is recommended. Live plants not only "eat" many toxic pollutants and freshen the air with oxygen; they probably slip in some extra negative ions as well!

NOTES

The human body operates on oxygen. Make sure yours gets enough by exercising, keeping your house well ventilated, and pausing frequently to take slow, deep breaths.

Air Inventory

Right now, without changing anything about the way you are sitting or breathing, answer the following questions:

1. How are you sitting right now? Is your spine straight, or are you slouching? Are your shoulders rolled forward?

2. Observe your breathing for a few moments. Is it shallow or deep?

3. Do the clothes you are wearing, or the chair you are sitting in, restrict your breathing?

4. Is the room you are in well ventilated with fresh air, or is it closed and stuffy?

5. Have you (or will you) exercise today?

6. Have you eaten a high-fat meal today? (A high-fat meal reduces your blood's ability to carry oxygen.)

7. When was the last time you got up and moved around? Have you taken a break or done some deep breathing during the past couple hours?

Breathe Deeply

Take a moment to try this simple breathing exercise. It will energize and refresh you.

Correct Breathing?

Place one hand on your chest and the other on your stomach. Breathe normally for a few moments, noting the movement of each hand as you inhale. Which hand rises more dramatically? If it's the one on your belly, take it off and pat yourself on the back. You have excellent respiratory technique. But if it's the hand on your chest, you'd better take a deep breath—though you probably can't. You're breathing wrong!

Stand or sit with your back straight. Exhale deeply through your mouth. Now, draw the air back into your lungs. As you do, imagine it going right down into your belly, filling it. Feel your stomach expand as you inhale.

When your lungs are full, slowly begin to exhale. Tighten the muscles of your stomach as you gently push the last bit of air out.

Repeat the process, slowly, five or six times.

Do this exercise when you wake in the morning and several times during the day. If possible, step outdoors into the fresh air. Refresh body and mind by giving yourself a caffeine-free boost.

Your Challenge:

Practice frequent deep breathing and experiment with other tips in this chapter.

Healthy by choice, not by chance!

NOTES

How Much Is Enough?

Tired of being tired?

Life today is fast-paced, exciting—and exhausting. Insomnia is epidemic. People are gulping down millions of sedatives and tranquilizers, desperate for rest that will restore their energies.

Why am I always tired?

You may have an illness, such as a cold or the flu, that is sapping your energy. Or you may be depressed.

Many otherwise healthy people, however, work in confining sedentary jobs with deadline pressures and emotionally draining problems. These people are not likely to feel rested when they get out of bed in the morning.

In addition, few people get through a day anymore without a pick-me-up, usually coffee, tea, or a cola. Caffeine is a central nervous system stimulant and a common cause of insomnia.

What about chronic fatigue?

Besides tiredness and a lack of energy, there is also an increase in irritability. Tempers get short, and patience goes out the window. Everything requires more effort, until finally the simplest tasks seem overwhelming.

Fatigue also sabotages creativity. Judgment suffers, and efficiency goes. And if unrelieved, fatigue can culminate in exhaustion and full-scale depression.

How does rest relate to these problems?

- Rest allows your body to renew itself. Waste products are removed, repairs are effected, enzymes are replenished, energy is restored.
- Rest aids in the healing of injuries, infections, and other assaults on your body, including stress and emotional traumas.
- Rest strengthens your body's immune system, helping protect you from disease.

> "And God . . . rested from all the work of creating that he had done."
>
> —Genesis 2:3

Proper rest can add length to your life. In a large population study of health habits a few years ago, it was found that people who regularly slept seven to eight hours each night had lower death rates than those who averaged either less than seven hours or who slept longer.

How much rest do I need?

People need different kinds of rest, and a relaxing night's sleep is a good start. Newborn babies sleep from 16 to 20 hours, while young children need 10 to 12 hours. Adults vary widely in their requirements, but most do best on seven to eight hours per night.

People also need a change of pace. During World War II Great Britain instituted a 74-hour workweek, but soon found that people could not maintain the pace. After experimenting, they found that a 48-hour workweek, with regular breaks, plus one day of rest each week, resulted in maximum efficiency.

Society also recognizes the need for other breaks from time to time. The long weekend is now an American institution and yearly vacations have proven their value.

Average sleep time declined 20 percent during the last century.

What about sleep medications? Are they helpful?

During normal sleep the body passes back and forth between periods of light and deep sleep. During light sleep dreaming occurs; this apparently provides a natural outlet for the pressures and tensions that build up during the day.

Medicated sleep, however, while producing a welcome state of unconsciousness, suppresses that dream stage. And even though people believe they have slept soundly,

they may not feel refreshed and energetic the next day.

In emergencies sleep medications may be helpful, but will contribute to chronic fatigue if continued over time. Others use alcohol to help them relax and go to sleep. But alcohol-induced sleep is not as restorative as natural sleep.

How can I sleep better?

- Take frequent breaks during the workday. Walk around, get a drink of water, take some deep breaths.
- Daily engage in 30 to 60 minutes of active exercise. Exercise relaxes, restores energy, helps banish depression, and combats nervous tension.
- Maintain as regular a schedule as possible for going to bed, getting up, eating, and exercising. The body flourishes on regular rhythms.
- Eat the evening meal at least four hours before bedtime. An

Did You Know?

- It's not only how much you sleep, but when and how regularly that matters.

- Fatigue is one of the most common of the complaints that propel people to the doctor.

- Teenagers need an average of nine hours sleep, but most don't get it.

- Some 70 million people have too little or very disturbed sleep every night.

- In a recent survey, 51 percent of men and 42 percent of women said they would go to sleep earlier if they didn't have television or Internet access. Being wired might make you tired!

The National Transportation and Safety Board estimates 100,000 car crashes causing 1,500 deaths and 71,000 injuries are caused each year by drowsy drivers.

The pace of modern society makes ever greater demands on us. But each week God gives an oasis in time that can help us find a new meaning in life for ourselves, our families, and others.

Some people overfill their lives just as others overeat.

empty, resting stomach is more conducive to quality rest.

- Try a lukewarm (not a hot) bath. It is a helpful relaxation technique.
- Count your blessings. Fill the mind with gratitude and thanksgiving.
- A clear conscience and a grateful mind are the pillows to sleep on.

Rest is an important part of life's rhythm. And like a dancer, if we go with our rhythms, we will be in tune with ourselves.

NOTES

"Come . . . to a quiet place and get some rest."
—Mark 6:31

Rest is an important part of life's rhythm. Most adults do best with seven to eight hours of sleep each night. If you have trouble sleeping, don't reach for sleep medications. Take a warm, relaxing bath. Exercise daily. Maintain a regular schedule. Strive for a clear conscience and tranquil mind.

Sleep Quiz

Feeling tired? Have a hard time getting out of bed in the morning? The following questions are designed to get you thinking about your sleep habits.

1. I have trouble falling asleep at night.
   a. Usually
   b. Often
   c. Rarely
   d. Never

2. I usually get enough sleep and awake feeling rested.
   a. Usually
   b. Often
   c. Rarely
   d. Never

3. I use caffeinated drinks (such as coffee and soft drinks).
   a. More than 10 cups/day
   b. 5-9 cups/day
   c. 2-4 cups/day
   d. Less than 2 cups/day

4. I go to bed at night early enough to get a good night's sleep.
   a. Always
   b. Often
   c. Rarely
   d. Never

Trouble Falling Asleep

Many people occasionally have trouble falling asleep. Three common reasons for this are emotional stress, caffeine, and lack of exercise. Fortunately, all of these can be controlled.

Caffeine, found in coffee, tea, and many soft drinks, can be reduced or eliminated from the diet.

Emotional stress can also be reduced by handling disturbing problems earlier in the day, when you are rested. Don't wait till bedtime to bring up problems.

A regular exercise program may be the best medicine of all for ensuring a good night's rest. It reduces stress and provides a pleasant physical fatigue that helps you sleep more soundly.

Getting Enough Sleep

For many, getting to sleep isn't the problem—making time for it is. Busy schedules, bolstered by strong coffee, cut into the hours needed for sleep.

Your body is your most valuable possession. It may be tempting to skip sleep, but in the long run that is counterproductive. A parable by Stephen Covey from his book *The Seven Habits of Highly Effective People* illustrates this point:

"Imagine you are walking through the woods when you come upon a man feverishly trying to saw down a tree. The man looks exhausted. He says he has been sawing on the same tree for five hours.

"'Why don't you take a break for a couple minutes and sharpen that saw?' you ask. 'It will cut faster.'

"'No time for that,' he gasps. 'I'm too busy sawing.'"

Here are some tips for getting some good shut-eye tonight:

- Go to bed and get up at the same time each day.
- Avoid caffeine.
- Don't use alcohol as a sedative. It makes the brain restless later in the night.
- Exercise early in the morning or late in the afternoon, but no later than three hours before bedtime.

The Ultimate Life

"I s this all there is?" sighs the aging baby boomer, surrounded by very considerable possessions. Having bought into the grab-all-you-can-get philosophy of the 1980s, boomers have every material thing their hearts desire. Yet they feel curiously empty and disappointed.

Isn't that a common human problem?

Yes, and it's getting worse. More and more Americans are living longer, healthier lives than ever before. Yet surveys show that they feel less and less satisfied.

Our hopes are continually being inflated by grandiose and unrealistic advertising, self-help gurus who promise the moon, and our childlike faith in medicine's ability to cure all of our ills. As disappointments pile up, we shuffle along looking for the missing pieces of our lives.

Are people ever really satisfied?

Early on we dream of wealth, fame, and success, of having what we want and doing as we please. But can you think of a multimillionaire athlete who isn't itching for a bigger contract? Or a wealthy celebrity who hasn't felt drawn to do yet another commercial, endorse a bigger product or produce a new book? Where is the business executive who wouldn't jump at the next big deal or lust after another merger?

On another level, do you know a teenager who is satisfied with his/her looks? clothes? friends? On the face of it, humans appear to be creatures of insatiable desires.

Is this why so many people turn to drugs?

In today's fast-paced life, people often feel so pressured and stressed, so full of pain and disappointment, and so hopeless that

"There is a way that seems right to a man,
but in the end it leads to death."
—Proverbs 14:12

they become increasingly willing to gamble their health and even their lives on almost anything that promises relief, no matter how temporary. "Follow your feelings," they are urged. "If it feels good, do it." "Hurry, life is passing you by."

For every skid row bum there are scores of closet alcoholics. And for every street punk looking for a hit, there are many so-called respectable people numbing their pain with prescription pills.

But lasting joy doesn't come in snorts, and well-being doesn't come from bottles and pills. You can't shoot up peace of mind. Gratitude and compassion aren't sold in the drugstore or on the street.

So where can I get joy, peace—those good things?

The Bible says that following our "fleshly" or "natural-feelings" leads to negative results like immorality, debauchery, selfish ambition, drunken orgies, fits of rage.

The Bible also says that God wants better things for us, such as peace, joy, and healing. These gifts, however, come through the cultivation of our spiritual nature.

Are such spiritual themes really relevant to life today?

You bet! Look at alcoholism, for instance. The medical miracles and the technological advances of the past half century have hardly

> A for-real relationship with the true God is never optional— it may be the very root of health.

touched this disease. Alcoholics Anonymous (AA) continues to offer the most consistently effective treatment with the best long-term results. AA uses a 12-step program that involves a recognition of human helplessness and the acceptance of a Higher Power. Similar 12-step programs, based on the philosophy of AA, are proliferating in almost every area of human need. They are bringing healing to thousands for whom medical care, drugs, counseling, and other human solutions have failed.

Today we are witnessing a renewed search for values, a resur-

gence of faith, and an increasing acceptance not only of a Higher Power but of a personal, caring God.

Could this be just another fad?

This so-called fad has strong roots in reality. One of the most exciting breakthroughs in recent years has been the discovery of the strong and close relationship of the physical, mental, emotional, and spiritual components of human beings.

This is a radical departure from the past. For centuries it was believed that body, mind, and spirit were separate entities that functioned independent of each other.

Now we're discovering that such things as anger, fear, resentment, and distrust can actually produce effects on the body that weaken its immune system and open the door to disease. Conversely, positive emotions, like love, joy, faith, and trust, produce protective substances that strengthen the immune system and protect the body from disease. Harboring bitterness and hatred, and nurturing negative thoughts and

Your Beliefs Can Affect Your Health

Weekly church attendance is good medicine. That's what Dale Matthews, M.D., of Georgetown University reports after reviewing more than 200 studies on the connections between religion and health. Religion has positive effects on patients dealing with drug abuse, alcoholism, depression, cancer, high blood pressure, and heart disease.

Trust in Divine Power

. . . means getting to know God well enough to trust Him for present and future well-being.

Whom can you trust?

Trust is like a bank account—if you build it up through daily deposits, it's there when you need it for an emergency.

Humans find focus, purpose, and meaning beyond creature comforts, needs, and desires through a relationship with God and adherence to His commandments.
—*Laura Schlessinger*

feeling, can make us sick; cherishing positive thoughts and feelings can make us well—literally.

What does cultivating my "spiritual nature" involve?

It could involve getting acquainted with that special Book, the Bible, singing praise songs, and praying for the special "fruit of the Spirit," such as—"love, joy, peace, patience, kindness, faithfulness, gentleness, humility, self-control" (Galatians 5:22, 23).

We are "fearfully and wonderfully made" (Psalm 139:14). We don't arrive in this world with only the minimal equipment needed for survival. We are each given a conscience to keep us on track; a full range of feelings and emotions to enrich our lives; and a brain that we can never use up or wear out.

Health and fitness are not enough. Neither are wealth, fame, good looks, or power. God has reserved a "special place" for Himself in every person's heart; as long as that space is vacant, everything this world has to offer will not fill it.

The ultimate lifestyle will be a life of spiritual growth that will supply the missing pieces and fill the empty spaces. The result will be a life of quality and fulfillment that will stretch beyond this life.

NOTES

_____

_____

_____

_____

_____

_____

"You will keep in perfect peace him whose mind is steadfast, because he trusts in you."
—Isaiah 26:3

Application

The ultimate lifestyle includes not just health and fitness; it also includes spiritual growth. Trust in God supplies a missing piece in our lives. It brings quality, fulfillment, and hope for the future.

Beyond Good Health

Good health is not the pinnacle of existence. Many who are otherwise healthy carry within themselves a deep longing for something more. At the root of our being is the need for greater purpose and meaning in life.

Poets and wise men have long affirmed this. Today even scientists are beginning to look into the spiritual dimensions of life.

Time

Like all things of value, cultivating the spiritual side of our nature takes an investment of time. Attention must be shifted from immediate concerns to deeper, more lasting issues. We need to take time for stillness, away from the commotion and noise of our everyday lives.

We need time to explore the deeper side of ourselves, to read inspiring words, or just to walk in the sunshine and fresh air.

When was the last time you allowed yourself to really enjoy the people closest to you? How long has it been since you joined with others who find faith and inspiration in a Higher Power?

We live today in a most exciting and yet paradoxical age. We can tune our radios and TVs to sounds and pictures coming from outer space or across the ocean. And yet many persons fail to tune their souls to God and to hear His voice.

The Spiritual Dimension

Where do you turn for renewal? What is at your core, your center of being?

Your Challenge:

Take some time to step back and think about what is truly important to you. Look beyond the clamor of daily activity to the universal themes of life. Choose an inspiring book, listen to some uplifting music, give thanks for the marvelous gift of life and health. Every breath you take is a miracle. Every morning is a new start.

> [Spirituality], then, is not a piece of information for the mind. It is a way of life, which includes all that we are, all that we do, all our hopes and aspirations, all the moments of our lives.
> —*Mario Veloso*

NOTES

_____

_____

_____

_____

_____

_____

_____

_____

People who have close ties to others, wh[o] share time and thoughts and worries and laughter with kindred souls, reap profound health benefits.

"THE RELATION that exists between the mind and the body is very intimate. When one is affected, the other sympathizes. The condition of the mind affects the health to a far greater degree than many realize. . . . Courage, hope, faith, sympathy, love, promote health and prolong life. A contented mind, a cheerful spirit, is health to the body and strength to the soul." —*E. G. White, The Ministry of Healing*

Mind-Body Connection

- ◎ Mind Power
- ◎ Depression
- ◎ Stress
- ◎ Endorphins
- ◎ Habit Formation
- ◎ Forgiveness
- ◎ Love

Our thoughts and feelings are the nutrition of our minds. Just as we need a certain balance of vitamins, proteins, and other nutrients for our bodies to reach maximum health and energy levels, we also need a specific balance of mental "nutrients" for a happy, tranquil, and creative mind.

You Are What You Think

Aristotle once said that a healthy body and a healthy mind were somehow intertwined, but the idea has traveled a rocky road ever since.

I thought that was pretty well accepted these days!

Yes and no.

Some scientists still question a direct link between emotion and disease, because they are not able to prove conclusively that a person's state of mind is able to cause or cure a specific disease.

What is emerging, however, is a better understanding of the body's immune system. While scientists can't take one particular emotion, such as anger, and relate it to a specific disease like a heart attack, they can now measure the body's immune response to specific stresses.

What is the immune system?

The human body is protected by millions of fighting units circulating in the bloodstream. These consist of different types of soldiers, each group having its own specific function. Central control can order out new units when disease invades the body. During times of peace the numbers are reduced, and the fighters become patrols. This is a simplified explanation of the immune system.

What affects the immune system?

A healthful diet, physical fitness, and positive emotional states can stimulate and strengthen the body's immune system. On the other hand, illness, drugs, and excessive stress can weaken it. AIDS occurs when the entire immune system has been decimated.

It may sound Pollyannaish, but staying optimistic in difficult times may keep you well.

"For as he thinks in his heart, so is he." —Proverbs 23:7, NKJV

Emotions can affect it?

Definitely. Scientists report that people in depressed and negative emotional states may be especially vulnerable to diseases affecting the immune system, such as asthma, rheumatoid arthritis, and cancer.

How can feelings affect health?

Some scientists call it the placebo effect. Perhaps the best way to explain it would be to illustrate it with a story.

Working late one night, I (Hans Diehl) was nearly overcome by sleepiness.

Remembering that my secretary keeps a jar of instant coffee in her desk, I added several tablespoons of the powder to a cup of water, gulped it down, and waited.

The immune system itself is an astonishing piece of work, rivaling the brain in its complexity and almost as difficult to track.

Within 10 minutes I felt energized—yes, caffeine mobilizes blood sugar. Then came heightened alertness—yes, it also stimulates the nervous system. I rushed to the bathroom, confirming that caffeine is also a diuretic. The boost lasted the three hours I needed to finish the project.

Next morning I confessed to my secretary. She listened and began to smile.

"I'm glad my coffee helped," she said. "But didn't you notice that it was decaffeinated?"

It worked because you thought it would work.

Yes. This placebo effect is commonly used to test new medicines. One group of test subjects is given the real thing, while another group receives the look-alike.

Nursing home patients who are allowed some say in day-to-day decisions, such as what food they'll eat, often outlive those who accept more passive roles.

◎

THE BODY grieves too. Rates of illness and death tend to be higher among those who have recently lost a spouse.

◎

A factor called "JOY"—meaning mental resilience and vigor—was the second-strongest predictor of survival time for a group of patients with recurring breast cancer.

Under Attack!

We are constantly exposed to and attacked by chemicals, germs, and viruses—so why don't these bad things overwhelm us? When our immune system is healthy and well, the bad things that attack us are fought off, and our health is preserved.

Surprisingly, placebo subjects often report results as good as, and sometimes even better than, the results of those who receive the actual medication.

In short, thoughts and emotions directly influence the mind, which in turn powerfully affects the body. On record are reports of people who believed they were going to die on a certain day and they did, even though no direct cause could be found.

Will positive emotions, then, strengthen the immune system?

Studies suggest that a stable emotional life is as important to good health as more traditional influences such as improved diet, regular exercise, and the avoidance of alcohol, tobacco, and other drugs.

Positive emotions and sensible health practices, it appears, can stimulate the production of endorphins. These mysterious substances are manufactured by the brain and can produce remarkable feelings of well-being. Apparently they pep up the immune system as well. Endorphins, in other words, help make you feel better while they also help make you well.

So I can cure myself by thinking nice thoughts?

You should never neglect whatever physical cures exist for a health problem. Giving up smoking, watching your weight, getting regular exercise, taking medication—all of these things are important.

But in addition, keep an eye on your attitude. As King Solomon said: "A cheerful heart is good medicine, but a crushed spirit dries up the bones" (Proverbs 17:22).

And Paul adds: "Whatever is true, whatever is noble, whatever is right, whatever is pure, whatever is lovely, whatever is admirable—if anything is excellent or praiseworthy—think about such things" (Philippians 4:8).

NOTES

Application

Thoughts and emotions directly influence the mind, which in turn affect the body. Research suggests that a stable emotional life is as important to good health as more traditional factors, such as exercise and diet.

Questions Are the Answer

We've seen that the mind and emotions have a powerful influence in our physical lives. But how do we harness that power to work for us? One answer is through the power of questions.

Questions Have the Power to Focus

A question is like a lens, turning the focus of your attention toward a specific problem or situation. When you ask yourself a question, your mind automatically goes to work looking for an answer.

The right questions can affect all areas of your life—relationships, attitudes, creativity, and ability to solve problems.

Five Powerful Questions

Here are five questions only you can answer. If you back up your answers with action, each of them can have a tremendous effect on your life. Be specific, and ask yourself the following:

1. What is the one thing I could do that would have the greatest positive, long-term effect on my life?

   _____

   _____

   _____

2. What is one thing I could do that would improve my relationship with someone I care about?

   _____

   _____

   _____

3. Ask this one often: What is there in my life, right now, that is worth being happy about?

   _____

   _____

   _____

4. What can I do today to develop a more healthful lifestyle?

   _____

   _____

   _____

5. Here's one to ask yourself when you are in a bind: If it were someone else in my situation, what would I tell them to do?

   _____

   _____

   _____

Don't Ask Yourself Negative Questions

Don't ask yourself such questions as "Why am I so dumb?" or "Why can't I stick to an exercise program?" Those kinds of questions focus your mind in a negative direction. Instead, rephrase them in a positive, productive way: "What can I do in the future to avoid this mistake?" or "How can I adjust my schedule to make exercising easier?"

Your Challenge:

Use these five questions and try to come up with several more of your own. You will be surprised at the power of this simple technique.

The Hopeless Feeling

Depression can be a serious, life-threatening illness—a major cause of suicide. Depressive disorders affect an estimated 30 million Americans throughout the socioeconomic spectrum, people of every age, race, religion, or education. Billions of tranquilizers and antidepressants are gulped down each year in desperate efforts to cope. Yet the problem grows.

Aren't feelings of depression a natural part of life? Don't most of us get depressed from time to time?

Feelings of depression are some of the most common emotions that humans experience. Depression is a normal emotion, but it can also be a symptom of a wide variety of medical and psychological illnesses.

Feelings of hopelessness and discouragement are frequently produced or exaggerated by the advertising media. Products that supposedly can magically transform people into capable, energetic, and happy new persons are presented. When this does not take place at once, many people experience disappointment and further erosion of self-confidence.

How do people know whether it's serious or not?

First, people need to understand the difference between discouragement and depression. Everyone is occasionally discouraged. Discouragement is a small dip in mood that good thoughts, prayer, and positive thinking can often lift. Discouragement usually has a defined cause, and is usually temporary.

Depressions are characterized by feelings of sadness and dejection, often accompanied by lessened physical activity. Feelings of unreasoning anxiety and a sense of hopelessness are often present. Let's look at some of the more common types:

- **The Blues**—The most common type of depression is often referred to as "the blues." A person may feel weepy, sad, discouraged, unable to cope, hopeless. These moods may be

Depression can appear suddenly for no apparent reason, or it can be triggered by stressful life events.

One of the most exciting findings of recent years has been the profound effects of exercise on emotional well-being.

brought on by excessive fatigue, excitement, or stress, or sometimes for no apparent reason. Such depressions are short and self-limiting. They rarely require treatment. People commonly bounce back to their usual selves in a few days.

- *Reactive Depressions*—These depressions typically result from intense life crises, such as losing a loved one or a job, going through a divorce, having children leave home, moving to a new location, or suffering a serious illness. At such times people are often unable to cope with their regular lives and responsibilities. A time of pulling back, of withdrawing, is needed to allow healing to take place. Supportive measures will usually take care of this, although more aggressive treatment may be needed if the depression is severe or prolonged.

- *Biological Depressions*—In contrast, these depressions come and go, usually with no discernible cause. They are often inherited, passed down in a family from parent to child. These depressions usually respond to treatment, although they may persist for several months despite treatment.

- *Somatic Depressions*—These more serious depressions usually interfere with adequate physical functions. Symptoms include problems in almost every system of the body, but they most commonly involve the gastrointestinal tract and the sleep cycle. Some individuals will deny being depressed, but their bodily func-

tions turn down, and their physical state has all the aspects of a depression. That's why psychiatrists call this a somatic depression—a depression expressed by altered body function: the body function is depressed even though the conscious mind may not be.

- *Psychotic Depressions*—These are depressions in which individuals lose touch with reality; they require professional care.

What can be done for depressed persons?

Nearly all depressions respond to basic, commonsense measures. For example:

- *Purposeful Tasks.* All of us need to do some kind of productive work, whether heading a corporation, washing a car, or cooking a meal. A depressed person in particular needs the feeling of completion, accomplishment, and satisfaction found in doing something useful each day. These experiences build on themselves, especially if the person receives recognition and encouragement.

- *Structure.* Whether depressed or not, we all need structure in our lives to keep mentally sound. Without something to get out of bed for, something to do, even the most stable person can at times become depressed.

- *Simple Diet.* Eating a simple diet of fresh, natural foods at regular intervals gives increased energy and decreases the physical stress of body functions. Depressed people especially should avoid concentrated sweets and heavy,

rich meals. Eating only fresh fruit for a day or two will do wonders in clearing the mind and banishing fatigue.

- *Adequate Rest.* Periods of quietness and calm are especially important in today's fast-paced pressured life. Chronic sleep deprivation can initiate or intensify depression. Most people do best when they get seven to eight hours of sleep a night. A few extraordinary individuals may need less, but even they must watch for signs of chronic fatigue. People who need more than nine hours of sleep are either unusual, ill, or convalescing. A person sleeping this much on a regular basis is likely to be depressed.

- *Daily Exercise.* One of the most exciting findings of recent years has been the profound effects of exercise on emotional well-being. Regular active physical exercise elevates mood, improves sleep, relieves stress, promotes health, helps to prevent disease, and increases the overall sense of well-being. The good news for depressed people is that the improvement in mood and attitude occurs through the release of endorphins in the brain. These "feel-good" hormones are activated by physical exercise. A brisk one-hour walk each day will do more good for many depressed people than medication.

Is there more?

Even severely depressed people can make simple everyday choices, such as deciding whether to get up in the morning or stay in bed; whether to watch television all day or look for more strengthening activities; whether to dress and groom themselves or stay in a bathrobe. Such simple everyday choices matter a great deal because they mold our capabilities for making choices tomorrow. It is by making good choices that people grow and become stronger. Even people with serious mental problems can improve their ability to deal more favorably with their life situations.

> A brisk one-hour walk each day will do more good for many depressed people than medication.

Encourage the depressed person to develop a list of goals. Write down positive and interesting activities. Then work on one item at a time. Checking each one off as it is done enhances the feeling of accomplishment.

> Regular active physical exercise elevates mood, improves sleep, relieves stress, promotes health, helps to prevent disease, and increases the overall sense of well-being.

People's attitudes and belief systems are at the root of all effective treatment. A person must understand that feeling bad or worthless is not the same as being bad or worthless. Feelings are temporary and they change, much like the weather.

To be worth living, life must have meaning and value. Otherwise a chronic emptiness and a fluctuating sense of despair may creep in and spread. We must, therefore, search to find reasons for living and codes to live by. This quest may lead to a progressive awareness of the reality of a God who cares about us. As spiritual growth takes place, it can bring answers to anxiety, fear, guilt, and resentment. And it can restore energy and release a new zest for living.

What about medical treatment?

Medications are frequently needed for psychotic depressions under professional care. Medications may also be indicated for certain biological depressions, such as bipolar affective disorders (manic-depressive mood swings).

Ideally, one should not need to take medication for emotional and psychological problems. At times when medications are needed, their use should be for a specific reason and for a limited time. Chronic use, especially of sedatives and tranquilizers, can lead to dependency and may actually deepen the depression.

Depressions that are unusually severe or last a long time need professional treatment. This treatment may include counseling, antidepressant drugs, or both. But even with professional help there are limits as to how much can be accomplished without the full participation of the patient. When people partner with their physicians, taking increasing responsibility for their lives, recovery can be greatly hastened.

Depression is no longer the dead-end, discouraging affliction it once was. By improving physical health, developing positive mental attitudes, making good choices, pursuing worthwhile activities, and developing spiritual goals and values, most people will be able to deal with their feelings of depression and live rewarding, productive lives.

NOTES

> "God has said, 'Never will I leave you; never will I forsake you.'"
> —Hebrews 13:5

Our health, happiness, and longevity, as well as our relationships with family, friends, and associates, and our spiritual life—are interrelated and interdependent. Improving our health, pursuing worthwhile goals, developing positive mental attitudes, and nurturing spiritual values can help us deal more effectively with our feelings of depression and hopelessness.

The Power to Choose

One of the things that sets us apart from other creatures is our ability to make choices. We can think about our actions, and we can choose between alternatives.

Family and Social Relationships

We are social creatures, and most of us do best when we experience a sense of community and belonging that comes from our relationship to others. When we feel isolated or in conflict, it is much easier to slip into depression.

A Higher Power

Through the ages millions have found comfort in time of need by turning to a Higher Power for strength and wisdom. Stories of people overcoming problems that seemed unsolvable are abundant.

It is easy for the hustle and bustle of life to crowd out time for spiritual nourishment. Yet those who have endured trying times can vouch for these values. Is your spiritual life the source of inspiration, strength, and renewal that it could be?

Here are some suggestions for boosting self-esteem and beating the blues. Write "OK" beside the ones that apply to you, and put a "?" beside those you would like to adopt.

_____ Look your best. Wear clothes that enhance your confidence.

_____ Play upbeat music.

_____ Speak well of yourself and others.

_____ Remember that you are unique. There is no one else like you.

_____ Make a list of your good qualities and focus on them.

_____ Realize it's OK to make mistakes.

_____ Consider a part-time job, a college course, an exercise class—a study group.

_____ Read self-help books. Take an "assertiveness" class.

_____ Go to a place of worship (even if you are not religious). Absorb the peacefulness.

_____ Play with a pet. Play with children.

_____ Take a long relaxing soak in your tub.

_____ Buy a surprise gift for someone.

_____ Clear up misunderstandings; don't let them fester.

_____ Relive happy times and remember pleasant memories.

_____ Help someone else.

_____ Nurture your spiritual life.

NOTES

_____

_____

_____

_____

Beating Burnout

If you removed the rocks, the brook would lose its song.

"Burned out." "Overloaded." "Exhausted." "Overwhelmed." These are some of the words we use to describe the impact of stress on our lives. In our time-pressured society, few escape without feeling—at least some of the time—that they are battling stress.

Stress has been linked with almost every medical problem we have—heart attacks, strokes, hypertension, ulcers, colitis, asthma, arthritis, even cancer. Yet too little stress can invite problems as well—fatigue, boredom, restlessness, low job performance, and depression. The challenge is to find a middle road between the two extremes.

What is stress?

Stress occurs in any situation that requires making a change. Most people define stress by problems that confront them and concerns they have to deal with.

Some stress, often defined as "eustress," can improve our awareness, promote alertness, and result in superior performances. Some examples might be sports competition, theatrical performances, skiing down a smooth slope, winning a race, receiving a job promotion. The stress involved in these situations can produce feelings of extreme pleasure.

Other stresses may not be quite so exciting yet cause strong feelings of satisfaction: a romantic evening, praise from a coworker, a child's good report card. Still other stresses may make us weary although they are good in themselves: a wedding, or a family reunion. Then there are stresses that exhaust and depress: a job loss, legal problems, rebellious children, divorce, the death of a loved one.

Health has been called the ability to adapt to life's stresses. If so, healthy people must find ways to pace themselves by keeping their stress in a positive balance.

Are stress problems getting worse?

The pace of modern life has thrown us into a kind of time warp. We are constantly urged to go now, see now, buy now, enjoy now. After all, as the ads tell us, we have only one chance in life, and we'd better grab all we can.

But after a few years of grabbing, getting, going, seeing, buying, we begin to feel battered and disappointed. The inevitable pay later comes along: burnout, debts, poor health, depression, and loss of interest in life. It's a vicious cycle that has trapped many well-meaning men and women.

What can we do about it?

To understand stress, we must recognize a critical distinction: the difference between "stressors" and "stress." "Stressors" refer to outside forces that we must deal with. "Stress" refers to the response of the individual to these stressors. We now know that it is not what we have to deal with (stressors) but rather how we deal with it (response) that dictates the severity of stress in our lives.

For example, picture a very cranky man walking to work in the pouring rain, cursing all the way. What is going on inside this man? Now picture three delighted children playing in the same rain. What is going on inside these children? Who has more stress? The difference is not in the circumstances, but in the attitude toward those circumstances.

EXAMPLES OF STRESSORS

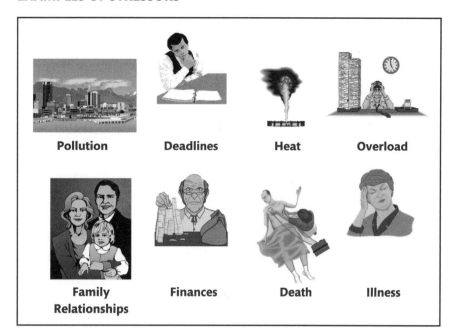

Pollution   Deadlines   Heat   Overload

Family Relationships   Finances   Death   Illness

To cope with the "distress" in your life, you must first recognize and identify the significant stressors you are dealing with. The awareness that the stressor and the stress response are not identical is critically important. So take time right now to list the 10 leading stressors in your life (on the Application page). Identifying these stressors opens the way for you to begin planning a process to cope with them.

Could you explain some of these coping processes?

There are many techniques that work, but here are some of the more important ones.

- *Healthy Adaptation* means that you recognize the stressor and do something positive about it. Ignoring or denying the problem is an unhealthy response, as is escapism.
- *Proper Planning and Organization.* These steps are required to deter-

Stress in the short term is vital, but over time it turns destructive. *Research is now showing how chronic stress breaks down the body and makes way for disease.*

Stress is the human response to overstimulation:

1. Sensory overload—noise, TV, lights, movies.
2. Information overload—TV, videos, newspapers, magazines, radio, computers, phone.
3. Decision overload—assaulted with 360 advertising messages a day . . .

—*Alvin Toffler, Future Shock*

> # God gave one day each week for:
>
> - **A weekly break from stressful living**
> - **Time for family and friends**
> - **Recharging your spiritual life**
>
> *—Exodus 20:8, 9*

mine what it will take to accomplish a task before you begin.

- *Positive Mental Attitude.* Don't be anxious about the future; take one day at a time. Worry tends to incapacitate, but seeing the problem as a challenge tends to motivate.
- *Committing to a Cause That Helps Others* and is approved by God. Isaiah 58 is one of the Bible's most sublime prescriptions for health.
- *A Healthy Lifestyle.* It's difficult to seriously damage a healthy body with stress. You can help protect your body against the harmful effects of stress with these simple stress inoculations:
  - ~ *Regular active exercise* for at least 30 minutes a day. Exercise produces endorphins, the feel-good hormones that protect the body against stress. Sunshine and fresh air also produce endorphins, so outdoor exercise is doubly beneficial.
  - ~ *A simple, plant food-centered diet.* The body easily handles such a diet. The result is increased energy, efficiency, and endurance.
  - ~ *No cigarettes, alcohol, caffeine, or other harmful drugs.* These substances all chalk up substantial pay-later debts, often beginning the next day.
  - ~ *Adequate rest.* This includes a good night's sleep and regular times for relaxation and recreation.
  - ~ *Liberal use of water inside and out.* Drink enough water to keep the urine pale (six to eight glasses a day). A hot and cold shower each morning starts your day off right.
  - ~ *Stable life anchors.* A spiritual center, a loving home, a job that makes you feel worthwhile, inspiring friends, a purpose for living—these are all vaccines against stress.
- *Thinking on Elevated Themes (see Philippians 4:8).* What we see and hear is under our control—movies, radio, TV, magazines, newspapers. Madison Avenue is successful because they use these mediums to focus attention on what we do not have, making us discontent. Remember: "The man who has little and wants less is richer than he who has much and wants more."
- *Trust in God* will provide a buffer against stress and a hedge against anxiety. Trusting God involves complete confidence in our heavenly Father to act on our behalf in the way and at the time that is best for us, according to His will.

As you can see, much of life does give us a choice. Don't procrastinate! Choose to enjoy life as it goes by. Praise the sunshine and the rain. Smell the flowers, return the smiles, play with children. This approach to life costs little and avoids hangovers. It exacts no pay-later debt. Instead, it pays generous dividends.

NOTES

Application

There are many things you can do to prevent stress from taking its toll. Regular exercise, a healthful diet, and stable life anchors all play a part in combating the effects of physical and emotional pressure.

Overcoming Stress

Too much stress is a very real problem in our society. Learning to deal with it has become an important health issue since studies began linking stress to a host of physical ailments. In most cases, running away is not the answer. We must develop more positive methods of coping.

Handling Overload

Sometimes it is possible to feel emotionally stressed without knowing why. When that happens, it is helpful to make a list of the things that are bothering you. Getting the sources of your stress onto paper allows you to focus and take action. Instead of overeating, overdrinking, or escaping into some time-wasting activity, you can identify the source of the problem and work toward a solution.

List Your Top Stressors:

_____

_____

_____

_____

_____

_____

What Can You Do?

Read these symptoms of stress, and check the ones that apply to you.

Do you suffer from:

☐ Increased irritability or impatience?

☐ Changes in sleep patterns?

☐ Changes in appetite?

☐ An increase in health problems?

☐ Difficulty in concentrating?

☐ Lack of energy?

☐ Lack of interest in things you used to enjoy?

☐ A sense of being "cut off" or isolated?

☐ A feeling of being "out of control"?

☐ Thoughts of suicide?

List three suggestions for managing stress that seem most valuable to you:

1._____

2._____

3._____

NOTES

....

....

....

....

....

The Happy Hormones

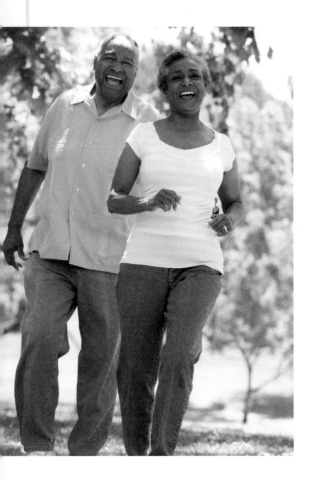

Happiness

is an inside job.

Feel-good drugs are almost irresistible. From cocaine to caffeine, people are reaching more and more for something that can help ease the numbing stress and paralyzing pressures that make up so much of modern life. But as evidence mounts that these drugs are destructive, scientists are discovering that a healthy body can make its own feel-good substances that are both protective and health-promoting.

You mean a person's body actually makes "drugs"?

Yes. If drugs are defined as chemical substances, then the body makes thousands each day. If drugs are defined as substances used as medicine to treat disease, the answer is still yes. The human body is engaged in constant efforts to heal itself.

What kinds of "good drugs" does the body make?

The most potent human-made feel-good drugs are the narcotics. Narcotics block pain and produce feelings of extreme well-being. They are valuable in controlling severe, unavoidable pain. Over time, however, they can become destructive and addictive.

Scientists have found that the body produces narcotic-like substances of its own. These can be lumped together under the general term *endorphin*.

Want to see these hormones in action? The next time you stub your toe or smash your finger, notice how quickly the intense pain fades and a comforting numbness sets in. People injured in accidents and soldiers wounded in battle seldom realize at first how badly they are hurt. Athletes can even fracture bones in the heat of competition and not feel the pain—until the game is over. These are examples of the body's endorphins at work.

Years ago Dr. Hans Selye found that fear or anger could trigger a blast of adrenaline in the body. The extra adrenaline produced a

> **"Whatever your hand finds to do, do it with all your might."**
> —Ecclesiastes 9:10

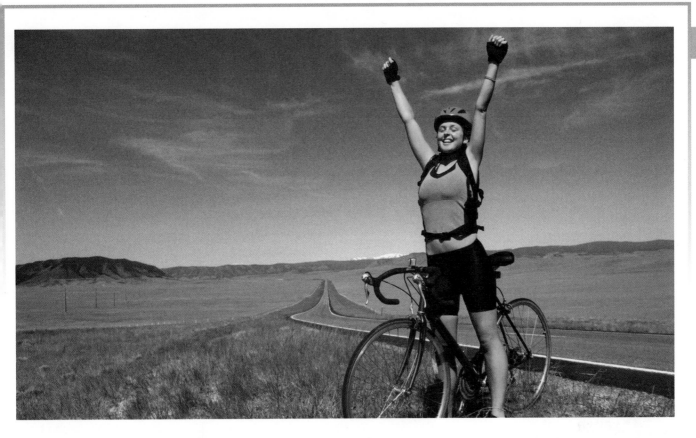

surge of energy that enabled the person either to fight or flee the source of danger.

Research later demonstrated that feelings of fear and anger can harm the body if they are experienced over long periods of time. Other negative emotions such as grief, hatred, bitterness, and resentment, if prolonged, can also exhaust emergency mechanisms and weaken the body's defenses against disease.

If negative emotions can be destructive, what about positive ones?

Norman Cousins opened the door to a new field of research when he helped heal himself of a fatal, hopeless disease by using positive emotions such as joy, laughter, love, gratitude, and faith, along with sensible health practices. Since then, scientists in the field of psychoneuroimmunology have isolated many of the substances these emotions produce in the brain. They are the endor-

He who has little and wants less is richer than he who has much and wants more.

phins. They not only block pain, but can also promote healing, strengthen the immune system, and produce wonderful feelings of well-being.

Are you saying that the way we think and feel can either damage or help heal our bodies?

Emotions are a very special part of our humanity. Clinging to persistent, negative emotions can promote disease, while nurturing positive emotions benefits every part of the body. For instance, physicians are learning that they must not shut the door of hope on terminally ill patients. The caring physician who, with confidence and optimism, tells a patient, "I have a feeling you are going to be that one person in 10 who conquers this disease," will often be surprised by a fulfillment of his prophecy. This is quite different from his saying, "You have only a 10 percent chance of surviving."

How else can we encourage the production of these special hormones?

We have known for a long time that physical exercise is beneficial to

How to Raise Endorphins

- Engage in daily active exercise
- Seek some solitude each day
- Be loving and kind to others
- Learn to say no
- Get enough sleep
- Don't procrastinate; plan your days
- Give away "stuff"
- Laugh a lot

health. But scientists began noticing that the good feelings that came from exercise could not be explained by their fitness effect alone. Something more was happening, and that something more proved to be an increase in endorphins.

Could this feeling just be a result of positive thinking?

The action of both narcotics and endorphins can be reversed by a particular chemical. A person whose pain is relieved with morphine will almost immediately lose that effect if this chemical is given. A person who is feeling a heightened sense of well-being from the body's production of endorphins will also lose that effect if the chemical is given. It's that specific.

But, yes, endorphin production is a result of positive thinking. Solving conflicts, banishing hatred and resentment, cultivating a loving, generous, thankful disposition, finding a strong faith—all these will boost the production of endorphins in our brains and strengthen the ability of the body to resist disease. And the physical benefit of a daily walk is the frosting on the cake.

The New Miracle Drug: Laughter!
Your whole body can benefit from a good laugh.

Advice From Scripture:

"Rejoice in the Lord always. I will say it again: Rejoice!"
—Philippians 4:4

"Do nothing out of selfish ambition or vain conceit, but in humility consider others better than yourselves. Each of you should look not only to your own interests, but also to the interests of others."
—Philippians 2:3, 4

"Our mouths were filled with laughter, our tongues with songs of joy."
—Psalm 126:2

"The fruit of the Spirit is love, joy, peace, patience, kindness, goodness, faithfulness, gentleness and self-control. Against such things there is no law."
—Galatians 5:22, 23

The body makes its own feel-good substances—endorphins—that are both protective and health-promoting. Physical exercise and a positive mental attitude boost the production of these endorphins in the brain and increase the body's ability to fight disease.

The Happiness Quiz

Part 1

It's easier to be happy when you feel healthy. Which of the following are you doing to boost your state of mind physically?

☐ *Exercise daily* (preferably in the fresh air): Studies show that exercise is one of the most effective cures for the blues. Certainly it is the least expensive.

☐ *Avoid caffeine:* Too much caffeine shortens your fuse and decreases your tolerance to life's stresses. It can also cause insomnia, robbing your body of much-needed rest.

☐ *Avoid Alcohol:* Alcohol is a depressant, yet many people turn to it during periods when they are experiencing negative emotions. That's like pouring gasoline on a fire. You don't need a depressant when you are feeling down.

☐ *Eat a low-fat, cholesterol-free diet:* Build it around whole grains, vegetables, legumes, and fruits. On this diet you will feel better, look better, and have more energy. All of these benefits create an environment in which positive emotions can flourish.

☐ *Get enough fresh air:* A well-ventilated house and frequent deep breathing helps keep your blood oxygenated. This is essential for being mentally and emotionally in top form. Fresh supplies of oxygen help keep you awake and alert.

Part 2

The mind and body are linked. Just as it is difficult to be happy when you are feeling the effects of physical illness, it's also hard to feel healthy when you are in conflict with yourself or others.

The following habits cultivate a happy, thankful attitude. How many of them are you developing?

☐ *Count your blessings:* Every one of us has much to be thankful for. Paying attention to what is good in your life rather than being overwhelmed by troubles is one key to a joyful existence.

☐ *Work toward harmony in relationships:* If you nurture the negative emotions of bitterness, envy, and jealousy toward others, you rob yourself of much joy. On the other hand, developing a forgiving, caring attitude brings happiness and friendship into your life.

☐ *Work for the good of others:* Reaching out beyond yourself to touch others helps you as much as it does those whose lives you brighten. Your emotional focus moves away from your own problems, and you feel good about yourself.

☐ *Take time for spiritual renewal:* The great men and women of all time have drawn strength and inspiration from their faith in something greater than themselves. This faith has helped them overcome obstacles and achieve greatness. Pausing from the rush of everyday life to contemplate the deeper things, reaching out to a power beyond one's self, may be the most effective means of bringing happiness back into your life.

Your Challenge:

Look back over the Happiness Quiz. Are there things that you aren't doing that might give your emotional life a boost? Choose one item; focus on it a few days—then make it a habit.

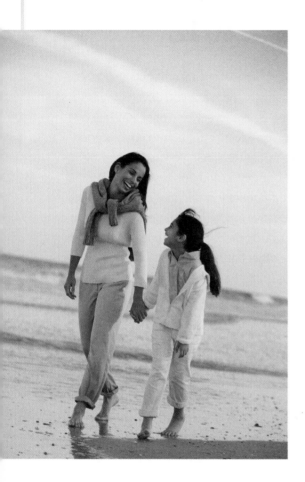
How to Change

Hard to get up in the morning? Hate to exercise? Can't shed those extra pounds? Most of us long to be different—to live healthier, more disciplined lives. Yet our most determined efforts to change too often come to nothing.

Why is it so hard to change?

Habits are what tie us down—and our lifestyles are often little more than the sum total of our habits. True, they can oil the machinery of our lives, helping us glide through our days, saving time and energy. (Who would want to have to stop and think how to tie a pair of shoelaces, after all?)

But habits can make our lives more difficult as well—and if you doubt that, try changing sides of the bed with your spouse tonight!

How are habits formed?

As you're probably aware, your brain sends messages to the rest of your body through nerve cells. Each nerve cell has a central processing headquarters and a long sending fiber (or axon) over which it relays messages. Nerve cells also have lots of tiny receiving fibers (or dendrites) for incoming messages.

Frequently used axons form tiny bumps; scientists call these bumps boutons, from the French word for buttons. And the more boutons a nerve cell has, the more easily and quickly it's able to transmit messages.

This helps us understand how habits are formed in the nervous system. Any thought or action repeated over and over builds little boutons on the ends of the affected axons, making it easier to repeat the same thought or action. It's almost as though the repetition wears a groove in the brain, much as repeatedly walking over

> *People are walking bundles of habits.*
> —William James

> The repetition of anything—good or bad—causes the habits to become confirmed in our lives: and fixed habits determine our character and our destiny.

the same place in a lawn will wear a path in the sod.

Once these pathways are formed, can they be changed?

Boutons, unfortunately, do not go away when they are no longer used. And because the old pathways are still there, the chance of falling back into a bad habit is always present, as when an alcoholic "falls off the wagon."

But people can change, can't they?

Yes, but only by building new habits that are stronger than the old.

The new choice must be made repeatedly, over and over.

That sounds tough!

It can be at first. But in time more boutons will appear on the new pathway than on the old one, and the "path" will wear deeper. As it becomes easier to take the new route, the new habit is being established.

How long does this take?

Most people find it takes about three weeks to form one new habit. A few years ago, for instance, a woman named Anya Bateman

Everything Changes!

I have a coin in my hand, and I give it to you. Now the coin is not the same! It is older, smaller (lost a few molecules), has a different temperature, there are different cells on it (from your hand), and its magnetic and gravitational lines have changed.

Living or not, everything in the world is undergoing change. You are constantly changing.

How you change is up to you.

How to Change

* You determine your destiny by the choices you make each day.
* How you think and feel shapes your character.
* Your choices actually make physical and chemical changes in your brain and nervous system.

decided to start flossing her teeth. What had been a tiresome chore, she learned, evolved into a bedtime ritual in less than a month. Encouraged, she applied her three-week plan to breaking her habit of eating too many sweets. Next she broke her habit of criticizing her husband, then formed a new habit of praising her kids.

By choosing our habits, we determine the grooves into which time will wear us.
—*Frank Gilberth*

The results were so astounding that they were published in *Reader's Digest.**

Likewise, just as some people become accomplished musicians by so many hours of daily practice, we can become a better person by consistently making good moral choices. And even if we lose a battle now and then, we won't lose the war—not as long as we get right back onto that new "path" we're trying to form.

So if you've always wanted to get some more exercise, try starting tomorrow. Get up a half hour earlier and hit the pavement with a brisk walk or jog. Sure, it may be tough at first—but in three weeks you'll have shed a few extra pounds, and you'll be on your way to a healthier lifestyle.

*Anya Bateman, "Three Weeks to a Better Me," *Reader's Digest*, September 1983.

"I can do everything through him who gives me strength."
—Philippians 4:13

Application

Why do good, strong, sensible people hang on to their bad habits when they know better? These people just grew into their habits while they were young, and now find it impossible to slip out of them. They are like a cucumber allowed to grow in a bottle until it is too big to take out.

Seven Lifestyle Factors

In the well-known Alameda County study, researchers followed 7,000 people for nine years. They were able to identify seven lifestyle factors that influenced how long people lived. They found a striking relationship between death rates and seven common health practices:

1. Not smoking

2. Exercising regularly

3. Either not drinking alcohol, or drinking only moderate amounts

4. Getting seven to eight hours sleep nightly

5. Maintaining proper weight

6. Eating breakfast daily

7. Not eating between meals

NOTES

_____

_____

_____

_____

_____

_____

_____

_____

_____

_____

_____

LIFE EXPECTANCY AND HEALTH HABITS

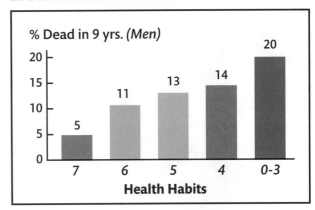

% Dead in 9 yrs. *(Men)*

Health Habits: 7 = 5, 6 = 11, 5 = 13, 4 = 14, 0-3 = 20

Findings:

- The fewer of the above health practices followed, the greater the likelihood of death.

- Only 5 percent of those who followed all seven practices died during the nine-year period.

- Some 20 percent of those who followed three or less were dead in nine years.

- Those who followed the greatest number of these health habits experienced only half the risk of disability as those with the poorest habits.

- Of men in the 60- to 94-year-old range, those who ate breakfast regularly and did not snack had half the risk of death of men who skipped breakfast and snacked.

Your Challenge:

- How many of these health practices do you follow regularly?
- Which ones are you going to adopt today?

The Key to Peace

New medicines come and go—but love has passed the test of time.

A touching story by Ernest Hemingway tells of a great quarrel between a father and his teenage son. Their relationship shatters, and the son leaves home. The father soon regrets the episode and goes in search of his son. But the city of Madrid is so large, so confusing—the father hasn't a clue where to look. He decides to put an ad in the paper. "Dear Paco, meet me at 10:00 a.m. tomorrow in front of the newspaper office. All is forgiven. I love you. Dad."

The next morning the father finds hundreds of Pacos in front of the newspaper office, searching, hoping . . .

That many young men longing for a father's forgiveness? That's heartbreaking!

Our world is full of hurting, heartbroken people—people who've been mistreated, neglected, alienated, victimized; people who are angry, resentful, bitter, lonely, depressed, fearful, and guilt-ridden; people consumed by hatred and self-pity.

But our world is also full of people longing for love, acceptance, compassion, and forgiveness, for someone to care, for spiritual comfort and peace of mind.

The spiritual hunger of people in this country is reflected in the skyrocketing sales of books on religion, spirituality, and inspiration. Recently one of the largest book distributors reported a cumulative growth in religion titles of nearly 500 percent over a two-year period. "This kind of growth for any category of books is unprecedented," he said.

Still, why are the answers so hard to find? Why do so many of us continue to live lives of quiet desperation?

One reason is that too many of us fail to realize that the cause, the root, of most of our problems lies within ourselves. For example, a wealthy, well-educated, but deeply depressed woman sought

> "Bear with each other and forgive whatever grievances you may have against one another."
> —Colossians 3:13

counsel. She suffered from recurrent headaches, ulcers, and obesity. "I'm bloated with fat," as she put it.

"He did it to me," she sobbed. Her husband, a respected politician, had had an affair. "I hate him for it, and I hate the woman even more. See what she's done to me? She's ruined my life."

The affair had occurred 13 years before, yet the woman remained obsessed with her bitterness and anger.

What then can we do for people who can't forget; when past pains refuse to be healed?

We could also ask What does their hatred do for them? To what worthwhile place does it take them? Why do they allow the hurts of the past to make a mockery of their lives today?

They need to know about the healing option. A painful memory is a mental wound, and they must let it heal. They must stop picking at the scab. They can't afford to keep an emotional scrapbook of their painful memories, because this is what imprisons them.

As the woman began to understand these principles, she realized how wrong it was to mortgage her present by clinging to her past. She needed to let the dead past bury its dead. SIt's been said that our attitude toward the past is far more important than the past itself. Attitude involves choice. What do we let life do to us—with its unfairness and its hurts? Make

us bitter? Or will we choose to let the difficulties in life make us better?

BITTER or BETTER? Are those the only options?

Studies indicate that people shown affection are less likely to see a doctor or feel sick. They also report a zest for life, love for work, and a sense that their existence is meaningful.

It pretty much boils down to that. Once a scientist watched a moth struggling to get out of its cocoon. It seemed that it just could not force its way through such a small opening. After watching awhile, he "helped" the moth by enlarging the hole. The moth emerged with a swollen body and shriveled wings.

It never flew. It needed that struggle through the small opening to force the fluid into its still-developing wings.

You're saying that we actually need hardships?

This world is a university of hard knocks. We owe it to life not to get bitter. Bitterness shrivels the spirit, causing spiritual atherosclerosis. Just as too much of the wrong kind of food hardens our arteries, nurturing the wrong kinds of emotions can harden our attitudes. Troubles, difficulties, and disappointments can push us to grow—in insight, in understanding, and in finding new directions for our lives.

Our depressed woman began to realize that she had to move away from her "poor me—pity me" attitude and begin to tackle her problems and learn to solve them.

"The moment I started to hate that woman," she reflected, "I began

FORGIVENESS

> We cannot change our past . . . we cannot change the fact that people will act in a certain way. We cannot change the inevitable. The only thing we can do is play on the one string we have, and that is our attitude. . . . I am convinced that life is 10 percent of what happens to us and 90 percent how we react to it.
>
> —*Charles Swindoll*

> It's what we value, not what we have, that makes us rich.

NOTES

to be her slave. For 13 years she has had a tyrannical grasp on my mind and my body. NO MORE! I know now that I can learn something positive from the most desperate situation. That woman will not steal my joy for even one more day of my life."

Basically, then, it was a change in her attitude that made the difference.

And a big difference it was! Here is another "attitude" story:

A high-society woman periodically checked into a luxurious suite of a New York hotel. She sought quiet time—to rest, to think, and to regain perspective. One time she heard a piano playing next door. Furious, she expressed her feelings in no uncertain terms.

The manager apologized profusely for putting Anton Rubenstein in the suite next door.

Rubenstein? The great one? The woman's attitude totally changed. She listened, she loved the music, and she treasured every day the renowned pianist was there. What had been noise before was now heavenly music!

A little understanding goes a long way!

Most of the time. One place many of us still stumble is over racial problems. Recently a popular Black columnist* for the Washington *Post* put the question in perspective by painting the larger picture. Here is a part of her editorial:

"I've felt hatred rage through me, washing away every barrier of reason and compassion. Hatred seeped through the crevices of my good sense, exploited the strains of my

Your Beliefs Can Affect Your Health

People who regularly attend religious services have been found to have lower blood pressure, less heart disease, lower rates of depression, and generally better health than those who don't.

- People who go to church have strong networks of friends who look out for them.
- Spiritual people are less likely to smoke, drink, and have other unhealthy habits.
- Taking part in prayer may lower harmful stress hormones.

everyday life, and chilled my compassion. Once hatred takes hold, it is hard to contain. When I'm in its grip, hatred can look sane and necessary. At such times I've screamed my loudest, cursed my rawest, and flailed away at my supposed enemy, until I'm exhausted; until I find my way back to love.

"Focusing too closely on hatred distracts me from a power more lasting and formidable—'the one power I can't afford to forget.'"

Beautiful! But aren't there some who do such horrible things that we shouldn't forgive them, much less try to love them?

It's easy to love the lovely people—what's hard is to love the unlovely. Mrs. Hannah's only child was raped and murdered by a man who was subsequently put in prison for life.

Mrs. Hannah hated this man intensely, and prayed that every day of his life would be even more miserable than hers.

One day "Gideon" (a man who supplies hotels, motels, and other public places with Gideon Bibles) came to her home and asked if she would care to inscribe a Bible for this murderer. She angrily refused.

Mrs. Hannah struggled on for weeks—for months. She finally realized she was trapped in her own prison of misery. There was no focus in her life, no joy, no triumph.

Finally Mrs. Hannah knelt down and pleaded with God to forgive her feelings of bitterness and hatred.

We cannot grow mentally, spiritually, or socially without practicing the grace of forgiveness.

Then the burden lifted, and she experienced peace.

She called "Gideon" and asked him to bring back the Bible—she was ready.

She opened the Bible and wrote—"Mrs. Hannah loves you." When the prisoner read this message, tears dribbled down his cheeks. He'd grown up an orphan. Never had he been told that anyone loved him. That one sentence changed his life. He trained to become a prison chaplain, and spent the rest of his life ministering to other prisoners.

And on that very day the old, bitter, hateful Mrs. Hannah died, and a new Mrs. Hannah took her place. She too realized she'd been imprisoned. It took forgiveness to set her free.[†]

At best we have a limited number of days in our lives. Isn't each day too precious to be marred by unforgiving thoughts?

Right on! Besides, do we really want to inflict on ourselves the pain and misery that we feel when we're not willing to forgive?

We need to ask ourselves—

Are there people I need to forgive?

Do I need to forgive myself?

People who learn to forgive suffer less anxiety and depression and have higher self-esteem. And they enjoy better health. A wise man said, "If you cannot forgive, you will live lonely, and the wine of life will be soured for you forever."

Love is more important than being right. Forgiveness opens the heart.

While being crucified by His tormentors, one Man prayed—"Father, forgive them, for they do not know what they are doing" (Luke 23:34).

To err is human, to forgive divine.

---

*Donna Britt, *Washington Post*
[†]Source of story unknown

NOTES

_____

_____

_____

_____

_____

The Ultimate Gift

*Someone's opinion
of you does not have
to become your reality.*

Mirror, mirror, on the wall,
Am I skinny? Am I tall?
Am I really who I see?
Do my friends know the REAL me?*
Perhaps you know yourself very well—know who you are and where you're going.
Maybe so.
Maybe not.
Probably not.

Why do you say that?

Because, deep down, most of us harbor feelings of low self-esteem. Although Americans now live longer, more prosperous lives, surveys show they feel less and less satisfied. We are increasingly a nation of whiners and hypochondriacs.

"If I could write a prescription for the women of this world," says James Dobson, "I would provide each one of them with a healthy dose of self-esteem and personal worth. I have no doubt that this is their greatest need."

Is it just women? Don't men have the problem as well?

Feelings of worthlessness and low self-esteem are certainly no respecter of persons. They cross lines of gender, race, age, color, and ethnic origin. People today are bombarded with overinflated expectations, grandiose hopes, and unrealistic representations of life. When their dreams fade and their hopes crash, when disappointments pile up, many become disillusioned and discouraged. Other people always seem to be doing better than they're doing.

They've missed out somehow. Life is passing them by.

> " 'Love the Lord your God with all your heart
> and with all your soul and with all your mind.'
> This is the first and greatest commandment.
> "And the second is like it: 'Love your neighbor as yourself.' "
> —Matthew 22:37-39

How about children?

Most problems with self-esteem have their roots in childhood. What happens during the first five years pretty much sets children's attitudes for the rest of their lives.

Many children grow up feeling unloved, neglected, and unwanted. They are yelled at and otherwise abused. Surrounded with too many negative messages and rules, they often become sullen, rebellious, hostile, and difficult to handle.

When they become teenagers, their feelings of worthlessness intensify. They long to be attractive, to be popular, or even just noticed. Their low level of self-confidence suppresses their talents and their personalities. The result is loneliness, isolation, perhaps bad relationship choices, and often drugs and prostitution.

That's a lot of bad news. Are there any good answers?

"When all else fails, try God." The phrase may sound trite, but the answers are there. God certainly didn't intend for any of us to suffer from low self-esteem. *"I have loved you with an everlasting love,"* He tells us; *"I have drawn you with lovingkindness"* (Jeremiah 31:3).

And the Master Teacher Himself, when summing up the great commandments, said that you shall *"love your neighbor as yourself"* (Mark 12:31).

Ultimate self-esteem comes from knowing who we are, why we are here, and where we are going. The Bible answers these questions in a beautiful and meaningful way.

- **Who are we?**
We are God's unique creation (Genesis 1:27). Among all the billions of people who have been born on our globe, there are no duplicates—not even among identical twins.

And that isn't all. We're told

that God *"knit [us] together in [our] mother's womb."* He knows when we sit down and get up. He understands our thoughts. Read for yourself Psalm 139, which spells out God's care from our earliest conception.

And the same God continues to love us unconditionally. *"Are not five sparrows sold for two pennies? Yet not one of them is forgotten by God.*

"Indeed, the very hairs of your head are all numbered. Don't be afraid; you are worth more than many sparrows" (Luke 12:6, 7).

- **Why are we here?**
To take care of the earth and its people, and to spread the good news of a God who is present and who cares about us (Genesis 1:26; Mark 12:31; 16:15).

- **Where are we going?**
God has told us that His house

has *"many rooms"* and that He is preparing a place for us to live with Him! (John 14:1-3).

And that's not all. He also promises that if we believe, we will *"have eternal life"* (John 3:16).

I'm impressed! God's plans and purposes for us completely upstage even the most spectacular of our human achievements!

Yes, and we need to help people understand what value each of us represents to our Creator. It's only when we realize this value that we gain true self-esteem.

The Master Teacher knew this. When we love ourselves, when we learn to fully appreciate this life God has given us, we can reach out to others—and learn to love them too.

Laura Schlessinger sums up this concept in one of her books: "People find focus, purpose, and meaning beyond creature comforts, needs, and desires through a relationship with God and adherence to His commandments." She continues, "For me it has meant a better and richer life, and a new significance in my work."

Do these concepts belong in a health book?

Obviously it takes a lot more than healthy food and regular exercise to make life worthwhile. People need dignity and respect. The need to love and be loved is as essential to health and well-being as are fresh air and clean water.

Too many people base their self-

> **Savor the things that bring you untarnished pleasure and satisfaction—food, friends, music, and the outdoors.**

LOVE

> **Most of us honestly admit that we seek a renewing purpose in life, a sense that life matters and that we can contribute something to the world.**

esteem on what other people think of them. But people's opinions are fickle, unstable, and certainly undependable.

Then there are people who are really in the gutter. They've been so betrayed, so rejected, so battered by life, that they cease to see any value in continuing the struggle of living.

But the Master Healer never passed by a human being as worthless, and we can't either. With a restored sense of self-worth, we become willing to take risks. And taking risks in loving others is what life is all about. "Dear friends,

- 'let us love one another, for love comes from God' (1 John 4:7);
- 'since God so loved us, we also ought to love one another' (1 John 4:11);
- 'let us not love with words or tongue but with actions'" (1 John 3:18).

Touch of the Master's Hand

'Twas battered and scarred, and the auctioneer
Thought it scarcely worth his while
To waste much time on the old violin,
But held it up with a smile.
"What am I bid, good folks?" he cried.
"Who'll start the bidding for me?
A dollar, a dollar—now two, only two—
Two dollars, and who'll make it three?"
"Three dollars, once, three dollars, twice,
Going for three." But no,
From the room far back a gray-haired man
Came forward and picked up the bow;
Then wiping the dust from the old violin,
And tightening up all the strings,
He played a melody pure and sweet,
As sweet as an angel sings.

The music ceased, and the auctioneer,
With a voice that was quiet and low,
Said: "What am I bid for the old violin?"
And he held it up with the bow.
"A thousand dollars—and who'll make it two?

Two thousand—and who'll make it three?
Three thousand once and three thousand twice—
And going and gone!" said he.
The people cheered, but some of them cried,
"We do not quite understand.
What changed its worth?" The man replied:
"The touch of a master's hand."

And many a man with life out of tune,
And battered and torn with sin,
Is auctioned cheap to a thoughtless crowd,
Much like the old violin.
A "mess of pottage," a glass of wine;
A game—and he travels on.
He's going once, and going twice,
He's going—and almost gone!
But the Master comes, and the foolish crowd
Never can quite understand
The worth of a soul and the change that's wrought
By the touch of the Master's hand.

—*Myrna Brooks Welch*

This is not a radical or new idea! Our health, happiness, longevity, and self-esteem—as well as our relationships with family, friends, and associates, and our spiritual life—are interrelated and interdependent.

How Much Are You Worth?

The story is told of a speaker who started off his seminar by holding up a $20 bill. In the room of 200 people he asked, "Who would like this $20 bill?" Hands started going up.

"I'm going to give this $20 bill to one of you, but first let me do this." He proceeded to crumple the bill into a small wad.

> **The worth of our lives comes not in what we do or who we are, but by whose we are!**

"Now who wants it?" The hands went up again.

"Well," he replied, "what if I do this?" He unfolded the crumpled bill and dropped it on the ground and started to grind it into the floor with his shoe. He picked it up, now all crumpled and dirty.

"Anybody want it now?" All the hands still went up.

"My friends," he said, "you have all learned a valuable lesson. No matter what I did to the money, you still want it, because it has not decreased in value. It is still worth $20."

Many times in our lives we are dropped, crumpled, and ground into the dirt by the decisions we make and the circumstances that come our way. We feel as though we are worthless. But no matter what has happened or what will happen, we never lose our value in God's eyes. Dirty or clean, crumpled or creased, we are still priceless to Him.

NOTES

_____

_____

_____

_____

_____

_____

_____

_____

_____

_____

"Pure air, sunlight, [temperance], rest, exercise, proper diet, the use of water, trust in divine power—these are the true remedies."
—*E. G. White,* The Ministry of Healing

"THE USE of natural remedies requires an amount of care and effort that many are not willing to give. . . . [But] those who persevere in obedience to [nature's] laws will reap the reward in health of body and . . . mind."

Coda

Basic Guidelines for a Lifetime of Good Eating

Eat Less:

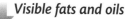

Visible fats and oils
Avoid fatty meats, cooking and salad oils, sauces, margarines, butter, dressings, and shortening. Use spreads and nuts sparingly. Avoid frying; sauté instead with a little water in nonstick pans.

Sugars
Limit sugar, honey, molasses, syrups, pies, cakes, pastries, candy, cookies, soft drinks, and sugar-rich desserts, such as pudding and ice cream. Save these foods for special occasions.

Foods containing cholesterol
Avoid meat, sausages, egg yolks, and liver. Limit dairy products, if used, to low-fat cheeses and non-fat milk products. If you insist on eating fish and poultry, use them sparingly.

Salt
Use minimal salt during cooking. Banish the salt-shaker. Strictly limit highly salted products, such as pickles, crackers, soy sauce, salted popcorn, nuts, chips, pretzels, and garlic salt.

Alcohol
Avoid alcohol and caffeinated beverages, such as coffee, colas, and black tea.

> "We cannot safely be guided by the customs of society. The disease and suffering that everywhere prevail are largely due to popular errors in regard to health."
> —E. G. White, *The Ministry of Healing*

Eat More:

Whole grains
Freely use brown rice, millet, barley, corn, wheat, and rye. Also eat freely of whole-grain products, such as breads, pastas, shredded wheat, and tortillas.

Tubers and legumes
Freely use potatoes, yams and sweet potatoes (without high-fat toppings). Enjoy peas, lentils, chickpeas, and beans of every kind.

Fruits and vegetables
Eat several fresh, whole fruits every day. Limit fruits canned in syrup and fiber-poor fruit juices. Eat a variety of vegetables daily. Enjoy fresh salads with low-calorie, low-salt dressings.

Water
Drink at least eight glasses of water a day. Vary the routine with a twist of lemon and occasional herb teas.

Hearty breakfasts
Enjoy hot multigrain cereals, fresh fruit, and whole-wheat toast. Jump-start your day.

COMPARISON OF DIETS (per day)

	Western Diet	The Optimal Diet
Fats and Oils	80-120 gm	under 45 gm
Sugar	35 tsp	under 10 tsp
Cholesterol	400 mg	under 50 mg
Salt	10 gm	under 5 gm
Fiber	10 gm	30 gm *plus*
Water (fluids)	minimal	8 glasses *plus*

Basic Guidelines for a Lifetime of Healthful Living

A checklist for making your new start:

Nutrition

- Nourish your body with healthful, full-fiber, nutrient-rich foods.
- Increasingly move toward a totally plant based lifestyle.
- Enhance digestion by breaking the snack habit.
- Schedule regular mealtimes, four to five hours apart.
- Eat larger breakfasts and smaller evening meals.

Exercise

- Strengthen your body and increase your enjoyment of life with daily active exercise, outdoors if possible.
- Aim for at least 30 minutes of exercise every day. Walking is the safest exercise and one of the best.
- Physical exercise reduces stress, combats depression, restores energy, improves sleep, and strengthens bones.

Water

- Rinse out and refresh your insides by drinking a glass or two of water on arising.
- Come alive with an alternating hot and cold shower in the morning.
- Lighten your body's metabolic load and increase circulation by drinking plenty of water—at least eight glasses per day.

> **"Through the agencies of nature, God is working, day by day, hour by hour, moment by moment, to keep us alive, to build up and restore us."**
> —E. G. White, *The Ministry of Healing*

Sunshine

- Pull back the drapes! Fill your home with sunshine! It will lift your spirits, brighten your day, and improve your health!
- Spend at least a few minutes outdoors every day.

Temperance

- Live a balanced life. Make time for work, play, rest, exercise, and hobbies.
- Nurture relationships and spiritual growth.
- Protect your body from harmful substances, such as tobacco, alcohol, caffeine, and most drugs.

Air

- Air out your house daily. Sleep in a room with good ventilation.
- Keep your lungs healthy by taking frequent deep breaths. Walk outdoors when possible.
- Fill your house with green plants that absorb carbon dioxide and increase oxygen.

Rest

- Reserve seven to eight hours a night for rest and sleep. The body needs this time to repair and restore the damage of daily wear and tear.
- Go to bed early enough to wake up feeling refreshed.
- Devote time to a change of pace. Attend church, go on a picnic, plant a garden, pursue a hobby, take relaxing, enjoyable vacations.

Trust

- A life of quality and fulfillment includes spiritual growth and development.
- Love, faith, trust, and hope are health-enhancing. And they bring rewards that endure.
- Trust in God augments all healing—physical, mental, emotional, and spiritual.

"Let Nutrition Be Your Medicine." —*Hippocrates*

To win the battle against the epidemic of Western lifestyle diseases, we must break with the lethal excesses of today's rich Western diet. We need a simpler, more natural way to eat, and a more balanced lifestyle.

As incredible as it might seem, there is one diet that not only prevents most of these killer diseases but also helps reverse them. Such a diet consists of a wide variety of foods "as-grown," simply prepared with sparing use of fats, oils, sugars, and salt. It contains very few refined, engineered products. Animal foods, if used at all, are strictly limited.

Adopting this simpler, more natural dietary lifestyle brings improved health and increased energy. We can eat larger quantities of food without gaining weight, and still cut our grocery bills in half. Where, indeed, can we find a better bargain than that?

"Many transgress the laws of health through ignorance, and they need instruction. But most of us know better than we do. We need to be impressed with the importance of making the knowledge we have a guide for our lives."
—E. G. White, *The Ministry of Healing*

INDEX

References

Abramson, John. *Overdosed America.* New York: Harper Collins, 2004.

Angell, Marcia. *The Truth About the Drug Companies.* New York: Random House, 2004.

Arloski, Michael. *Wellness Coaching for Lasting Life Change.* Duluth, MN: Whole Person Assoc., 2007.

Barnard, Neal. *Eat Right, Live Longer.* New York: Harmony Books, 1995.

Barnard, Neal. *Dr. Neal Banard's Program for Reversing Diabetes.* New York: Rodale, 2007.

Barnard, Neal. *Nutrition Guide for Clinicians.* Washington, DC: PCRM, 2010.

Barnard, Neal. 21-day *Weight Loss Kick Start.* New York: Grand Central Life of Style, 2011.

Buettner, Dan. *The Blue Zone.* Washington, DC: National Geographic Society, 2008.

Campbell, T. Colin and Thomas. *The China Study.* Dallas, TX: BenBella Books, 2005

Esselstyn, Caldwell. *Prevent and Reverse Heart Disease.* New York: Penguin Group, 2008.

McDougall, John. *A Challenging Second Opinion.* New York: Penguin Books.

Messina, Virginia. *The Vegetarian Way.* New York: Crown, 1996.

Nedley, Neil. *Proof Positive.* Ardmore, OK: Nedley Publishing, 1998.

Nedley, Neil. *The Lost Art of Thinking.* Nedley Publishing. 2011.

Nelson, Ethel. *Burkitt—Cancer, Fiber— How a Humble Surgeon Changed the World.* Brushton, N.Y.: TEACH Services, 1998.

Ornish, Dean. *Dr. Dean Ornish's Program for Reversing Heart Disease.* New York: Random House, 1990.

Robbins, John. *Reclaiming Our Health.* Tiburon, Calif.: H. J. Kramer, 1996.

Steale, Stuart. The Full Plate Diet. Austin, TX: Bard Press, 2010.

Thompson, Walter. *Health Smart.* W. Frankfort, IL: 3ABN Books, 2010.

Weber, Karl. Food Inc. Philadelphia: Perseus Book Grouup, 2009.

White, E. G. *The Ministry of Healing.* Nampa, Idaho: Pacific Press, 1909.

Are you ready to take the next step?

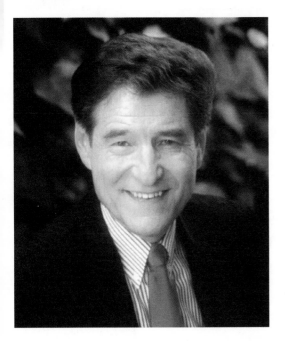

Then look for the CHIP program nearest you and enroll! Take 30 days—and change your life and health forever!

What's CHIP?

CHIP is an educationally intensive 30-day lifestyle intervention program with more than 50,000 graduates. Founded by Hans Diehl, the program and its clinical results have been published in more than 20 peer-reviewed medical journal articles. Endorsed by the Physicians' Committee for Responsible Medicine and the Center for Science in the Public Interest, the Coronary Health Improvement Project (CHIP) focuses on markedly reducing coronary risk factors through the adoption of better health habits and wiser lifestyle choices.

What will it do for me?

Overweight? It will show you how to eat more and still lose all the weight you want. *Hypertension?* It will lower your blood pressure and your medication needs. *Diabetes (type 2)?* It will help you to lower your blood sugar and your medication requirements. *Cholesterol?* CHIP will bring your elevated cholesterol down on average 10-20 percent without medication. *Heart disease?* It will show you how to slow down, halt, and facilitate the reversal of coronary artery disease. *Depression?* It will give you the lift and energy you've been looking for.

Where can I find CHIP?

CHIP programs are conducted in more than 250 locations in North America—in cities, corporations, and churches. For more information, please call the Lifestyle Medicine Institute at: **909-796-7676**, or online at: www.CHIPonline.orgg. We'll be looking forward to helping you with your new journey.

Special life-saving resources... www.CHIPonline.org

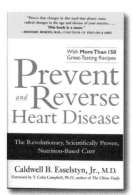

Prevent & Reverse Heart Disease
by Caldwell B. Esselstyn, Jr., MD, Cleveland Clinic

Based on the groundbreaking results of his 20-year nutritional study, Dr. Esselstyn explains, with irrefutable scientific evidence, how we can end the heart disease epidemic in this country by changing what we eat. Backed by real science, startling angiograms, and inspiring personal stories, this book is a powerful call for a paradigm shift in coronary artery disease therapy. After all, expensive surgical procedures and drugs fail to be effective over time, and they are dangerous to patients.

Dr. Diehl Health Seminar Set
Filmed at the Gaylord Hotel in Dallas, TX at the Dr. Errol Bryce Health Seminar, Dr. Diehl delivered these two keynote addresses.

Lifestyle Medicine: Its Time Has Come
Dr. Hans Diehl spells out with startling clarity in this 75-min. presentation the role of lifestyle in matters of health. You will be convinced that health, and even healthcare, is now in our hands. Medicine is no longer the lord of our well-being.

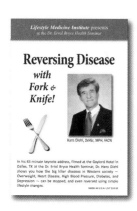

Reversing Disease with Fork & Knife
Dr. Hans Diehl shows you in this 65-min. presentation how the big killer diseases in Western society — Overweight, Heart Disease, High Blood Pressure, Diabetes, and Depression — can be stopped, and even reversed using simple lifestyle changes.

The China Study
by T. Colin Campbell, PhD & Thomas Campbell

The most comprehensive study in nutrition ever conducted! A landmark release demonstrating the definite advantages of a more natural diet over the rich Western dietary lifestyle. Plus, a disturbing look behind the scenes of the world of science. Bestseller: over 500,000 copies in circulation. 418 pp.

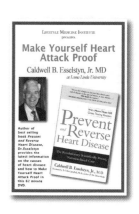

"Written with candor, courage and clarity, and with intellectual honesty and profound insight, this compelling book could become the national tipping point towards contagious health!"

--Hans Diehl, DrHSc, MPH

Make Yourself Heart-Attack Proof
by Caldwell Esselstyn, Jr, MD

Filmed at Loma Linda University, Dr. Esselstyn (Cleveland Clinic) provides in this 62-min. DVD the latest information on the causes and cure for Coronary Artery Disease. You will be inspired.

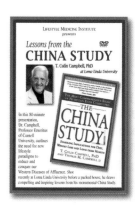

Lessons from the China Study
by T. Colin Campbell, PhD

Filmed at Loma Linda University, Dr. T. Colin Campbell (Professor Emeritus, Cornell University) outlines in this 80-min. powerful presentation the need for a new lifestyle paradigm to reduce and conquer our Western Diseases of Affluence.

www.CHIPonline.org

www.vibrantlife.com

Vibrant life

mind — *body* — *spirit*

www.VibrantLife.com

vibrant life.

America's First Health Magazine

Achieve a Healthy Mind, Body, and Spirit

▸ Two Words that Can Change Your Life

▸ How to Improve Your E.Q.

▸ 21 Tips for Spiritual Growth

▸ Healthy Recipes in 3 Steps or Less

Forks Over Knives

An exclusive interview with Dr. T. Colin Campbell, author of *The China Study,* and Dr. Caldwell Esselstyn, stars of the new blockbuster movie.

Could you do a marathon a day for 100 days?

Leo Schreven, 50, attempts the incredible!

0 74470 19180 0   05   May/June 2011

If you're determined to live a healthier and more energetic life, we're here to support you. Every issue of *Vibrant Life* encourages you to keep choosing better foods to eat. It provides vegetarian recipes that will attract the whole family. There's good advice on finding exercises that fit your lifestyle and natural remedies for the aches and pains that slow you down. *Vibrant Life* helps you stay on track--mentally, physically, and spiritually.

K20-01-0

Call (800) 456-3991 or order online at: www.VibrantLife.com